TREAT THEM WHERE THEY LIE

Pioneering a Revolution in Modern Emergency Medicine

A Memoir by

Dr. Ron Stewart
with Jim Meek

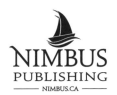

NIMBUS
PUBLISHING
— NIMBUS.CA —

Nimbus Publishing Limited
3660 Strawberry Hill Street, Halifax, NS, B3K 5A9
(902) 455-4286 nimbus.ca

Printed and bound in Canada

NB1748
Editor: Angela Mombourquette
Cover photo: Michael Creagan
Cover design: Heather Bryan

Nimbus Publishing is based in Kjipuktuk, Mi'kma'ki, the traditional territory of the Mi'kmaq People.

Library and Archives Canada Cataloguing in Publication

Title: Treat them where they lie : pioneering a revolution in modern emergency
    medicine / a memoir by Dr. Ron Stewart with Jim Meek ; forewords by
    Dr. Brian Goldman, Dr. Brian Zink.
Names: Stewart, Ronald D., author. | Meek, Jim, 1950- author.
Description: Includes index.
Identifiers: Canadiana (print) 20240364791 | Canadiana (ebook)
    20240364929 | ISBN 9781774713105 (softcover) |
    ISBN 9781774713150 (EPUB)
Subjects: LCSH: Stewart, Ronald D. | LCSH: Emergency physicians—
    Canada—Biography. | LCSH: Emergency physicians—United States—
    Biography. | LCSH: Legislators—Nova Scotia—Biography. | LCSH:
    Emergency medicine. | LCGFT: Autobiographies.
Classification: LCC RA975.5.E5 S74 2024 | DDC 616.02/5092—dc23

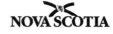 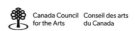

Nimbus Publishing acknowledges the financial support for its publishing activities from the Government of Canada, the Canada Council for the Arts, and from the Province of Nova Scotia. We are pleased to work in partnership with the Province of Nova Scotia to develop and promote our creative industries for the benefit of all Nova Scotians.

Dedicated to the courageous men and women who serve as first responders in all parts of the world.

CONTENTS

A CAREER IN THREE ACTS

A FAIR NUMBER OF COLLEAGUES ASK ME TO WRITE A BLURB THAT SINGS THE PRAISES OF their work. In general, I'm happy to do it because doing so validates their authorship. Occasionally, I'm asked to write a foreword to the book. It takes more work, and I have no time for extra work. That said, there are some colleagues to whom you cannot say no.

Dr. Ronald Stewart is one such colleague. Ron is so accomplished that I could never be in his league. Not that he sees it that way, as he revealed in an email he sent to me some months before the formal request came to write the foreword.

"Hello from the Cape Breton woods, Brian," he wrote to me. "I continue to feel still very much connected with you. Not via any frequent correspondence but rather via my being a faithful listener and admirer of the fantastic medicine you practice over the airwaves. I am hoping you realize the depth and breadth of your influence-for-good you've exercised over the years. I have both admired and envied what you're doing and happily think frequently to myself 'I knew him when.'"

That paragraph suits Ron perfectly. He is an incredibly accomplished man who, despite accomplishing great things, never sees himself as being greater than a neighbour, patient, or colleague like me. Then as now, Ron remains humble and curious. These are character traits that ring true in the memoir you are about to read.

Ron was born in North Sydney, Nova Scotia, and was raised in Sydney Mines. The son of a coal miner, early on, he developed empathy for workers who were exploited without benefits. He sang in a local church choir and eventually learned to play the bagpipes.

Ron's interest in medicine started early. As a draegerman, his father was trained in first aid and other mine rescue techniques. Sensing Ron's budding fascination, his dad fashioned him an age-appropriate first aid kit. Ron never looked back. He got his BA and BSc degrees from Acadia University before obtaining his medical degree at Dalhousie University in 1970.

He had a strong interest in emergency medicine that began during a rotation in the ER at Victoria General Hospital under the tutelage of Dr. Robert Scharf, a general and orthopedic surgeon who served as the hospital's head of emergency medicine. Tellingly, Scharf organized the first clinical courses for ambulance attendants in Nova Scotia.

At the time, emergency medicine as a specialty was in its infancy. There were very few widely respected residency training programs in the United States, let alone in Canada. Instead, Ron followed his rotating internship by starting general practice in Neils Harbour in northern Cape Breton. Call that Act One of his medical career.

It took a horrific accident to spur him to pivot back to his first love. He was on a house call during a severe snowstorm when his car plunged over a cliff near Neils Harbour. It was 3:00 A.M., and he was fortunate to be rescued. Following a long recovery, Ron returned to general practice and quickly discovered that, while his ability to care for his patients had not been affected, his patients were uncomfortable with his speech challenges. As he writes in the book, his patients took to finding out which hours and days he worked so they could book appointments with his associate instead. Ron felt this situation was unfair to his partner, so he arranged for a new partner to join the practice and then headed off to a residency (after intensive speech therapy) in LA. It's brave and humble of Ron to share such a frank observation with us.

Good people become great by rebounding from challenges. The circumstances of Ron's switch from general practice to emergency medicine resonates with me personally. During medical school, I had every intention to become a pediatric neurologist. As part of my plan to win a coveted residency position in the US, I did a two-month elective in neurology at Johns Hopkins Hospital in Baltimore. My pivot was not precipitated by a severe head injury but by sleep deprivation. The morning I was scheduled to present grand rounds in the Department of Neurology, I slept in, and thus missed my one and only opportunity to impress my neurology mentors.

What felt to me at the time like an unfortunate episode became an opportunity to change direction. Returning to Toronto, I realized that I loved writing and broadcasting as much as I loved medicine. Being an ER physician enabled me to do both.

In 1972, Ron won a coveted residency in emergency medicine at Los Angeles County/USC (LAC+USC) Medical Center. He was chosen over fifty-nine other applicants. His early experiences treating gang members who suffered gunshot wounds taught him how emergency physicians can stabilize patients so they make it to the operating room where surgeons can then perform damage-control surgery. He also became a script consultant on the hit American TV show, *Emergency!* There, he helped authenticate a fictionalized version of paramedics pulling patients back from the brink.

In 1979, he left LA to become the founding head of the emergency medicine department at the University of Pittsburgh. There, he built a powerhouse residency in emergency medicine and helped make the idealized TV version of paramedicine a reality. Call that Act Two of his career as a builder of emergency medicine.

In 1988, Ron returned to Canada, making a pitstop in Toronto as an emergency physician and (briefly) head of the trauma unit and the air ambulance service at Sunnybrook Health Sciences Centre.

That he spends but three pages of the book chronicling his proverbial "cup of coffee" in Toronto gives a strong clue that it wasn't a happy time for him. Like general practice in Cape Breton, one can argue that Ron and Sunnybrook weren't right for one another.

Once again, Ron pivoted to a greater destiny. In 1989, he returned to Nova Scotia. Just four years later, he entered provincial politics, defeating Progressive Conservative cabinet minister Brian Young in the riding of Cape Breton North. In June 1993, he was appointed minister of health. Act Three was underway.

As health minister, Ron played a major role in reforming Nova Scotia's healthcare system. Under his stewardship, in 1994, the province took control of various antiquated ground ambulance operations and consolidated them into a single entity called Emergency Health Services.

Once again, he rebounded from disappointment to a much greater level of achievement.

Think of that lesson as you read about Ron's incredible career.

– Dr. Brian Goldman

DR. BRIAN GOLDMAN IS AN EMERGENCY PHYSICIAN IN TORONTO AND THE HOST OF *WHITE COAT, BLACK ART* ON CBC RADIO ONE. HE IS THE AUTHOR OF FOUR CANADIAN NON-FICTION BESTSELLERS. HIS LATEST, *THE POWER OF TEAMWORK: HOW WE CAN ALL WORK BETTER TOGETHER*, WAS PUBLISHED IN 2022.

IT STARTS IN THE STREET

THE FIELD OF EMERGENCY MEDICINE ATTRACTS MANY PHYSICIANS WITH INTERESTING backgrounds, but Dr. Ronald Stewart's life history is unique and intriguing. It also extends well beyond the bounds of clinical medicine.

I first met Ron in 1983 when I was an emergency medicine residency applicant and had travelled to the University of Pittsburgh to interview at the new but highly regarded residency program Ron started. I didn't get the chance to talk much with Ron. Just as we sat down to the interview, a pager went off and I was whisked away by a resident to bounce over the hilly streets of Pittsburgh in a Ford Bronco in response to an emergency medical services (EMS) call. This was one of Ron's innovations—shortly after starting the program at the university, he secured the vehicles needed to get emergency medicine residents directly involved in EMS care. He knew effective emergency care had to start in the street—a lesson he'd learned as an emergency medicine resident in the pioneering program at the University of Southern California in Los Angeles County. This was a lesson he also applied in his creative and energetic development of what would become the legendary Los Angeles County paramedic training program.

As I progressed in my academic career, I was aware of Ron's continued success in building an academic emergency medicine powerhouse at Pittsburgh, which also became a major research centre under his leadership. I saw him speak at our national academic meetings, but didn't get to know him well until 2002, when I embarked on a three-year project to write a comprehensive modern history of US emergency medicine.[1] I sought first-hand sources, determined to travel the continent while I was on sabbatical from the University of Michigan to complete oral history interviews with founders of the field. I knew that Ron had returned to his native Nova Scotia and I emailed him, hoping to perhaps connect with him at a national emergency medicine conference in the US. Then I experienced Ron's generosity and kindness—he invited me (and my wife and three kids) to Nova Scotia to stay at his Annex House on Boularderie Island. He also promised us a personal tour of his beloved Cape Breton. I couldn't refuse that kind offer. The experience was memorable. I interviewed Ron with my old Sony analog tape recorder sitting between us on the kitchen table of the compact cliffside bungalow that he and his father had built on forested land overlooking the Great Bras d'Or Channel. A bald eagle flew by the window. Ron related many of the stories that appear in this book—but far too many for me to include in mine. I was laughing, shaking my head—entranced by the life journey of this coal miner's son.

And then there was the tour. We set off early in the morning and drove around the island of Cape Breton, with Ron in the front seat narrating every kilometre like an affable tour guide. We made stops in small fishing towns, nature areas, and at Ron's favourite eateries. During this journey, my understanding of Ron Stewart was transformed. Experiencing his deep, spiritual connection to that beautiful land and his unabashed love for the place and its people took me beyond "Dr. Stewart—emergency medicine pioneer and EMS leader, educator, mentor"—to "Ron Stewart, community builder, philosopher, politician, musician, naturalist, and beloved friend of Nova Scotia." We stopped at the home of friends, harvested and ate oysters out of the bay, and chatted with EMS crews at a coffee shop. Ron showed us nursing homes to which he had brought a medical student a cappella group from Dalhousie to sing for seniors. Everywhere we stopped, the affection, respect, and admiration that the people of Cape Breton had for Ron was palpable. I came to appreciate that this man, who was immensely important to the establishment of emergency medicine and EMS during his eighteen years in the US, was just as important to his homeland of Nova Scotia, but in a different, granular, deep-rooted way. In his tenure as his home province's minister of health in the 1990s, he had introduced a modern EMS system (no longer do hearses do double duty as ambulances in rural areas).

Ron Stewart's impact on the realm of emergency medical services (EMS) in North America, and even around the world, has been profound. Starting with his key role in training the first paramedics in Los Angeles County, and then serving as advisor to the 1970s television show *Emergency!*, Ron's ability to look beyond what is and to see what is possible has been evident in every step of his journey. He put emergency medicine residents in the streets of Pittsburgh. He recognized the need for a national organization to build and guide the field of EMS and co-founded the National Association of EMS Physicians (NAEMSP), serving as its first president. After he returned to Nova Scotia, Ron became a vocal, passionate, and effective advocate of the progressive anti-smoking legislation Canada's national government passed in 1997. As a leader in the World Association for Emergency and Disaster Medicine (WADEM), he wrote the anti–land mines resolution that the organization's membership unanimously endorsed, and he presented it to the 1997 United Nations conference that ratified the global treaty to eliminate the use of land mines.

One of the goals I had in writing the first comprehensive modern history of US emergency medicine was to bring the personal stories of its founders to light. One of the frustrating aspects of that project was that there was not enough "room" to include more details from the hours of interviews I conducted. In this memoir, Ron Stewart and Jim Meek provide the details and insights of a life that deserves to be fully chronicled and understood. Not that Ron's ego needs this exposure—his modest, self-deprecating nature does not seek more acclaim. (This memoir barely mentions his honorary degrees or catalogue of awards, nor does it dwell on his academic publications, though there were dozens of them.) In short, Ron Stewart is one of a kind whose life has been about helping all of our kind. The value of this memoir, then, is for the rest of us to see how passion, a dogged pursuit of what is right, and a creative, even quirky, spirit for innovation and taking chances can lead to so many positive changes that benefit society.

– Dr. Brian Zink

DR. BRIAN ZINK IS A PROFESSOR OF EMERGENCY MEDICINE AT THE UNIVERSITY OF MICHIGAN AND THE AUTHOR OF *ANYONE, ANYTHING, ANYTIME: A HISTORY OF EMERGENCY MEDICINE.*

LOS ANGELES, 1974

MY PATIENTS WERE DYING IN THE CITY STREETS BUT LIVING ON THE TV SCREENS IN people's homes.

Let me explain. My day job was training a new generation of paramedics in Los Angeles. That work took me into people's homes, down dark alleys, and onto freeways, alongside firefighters and other first responders who treated victims of heart attacks, drug overdoses, gunshot wounds, and automobile crashes. My "Doc Hollywood" gig was acting as a script- and occasional on-set advisor for the TV series *Emergency!*, a hit show in which accident victims played by actors had a much better chance of surviving than their real-life counterparts in the city.

In the 1970s, EMS systems were in their infancy. On television, though, the medics and physicians were competent (and handsome), the nurses were compassionate (and beautiful), and nearly dead patients were routinely brought back to life. Real life was starkly different, as you'll learn in this memoir. Patients, including Bobby Kennedy on the night of his assassination in 1968, were sometimes taken to an inappropriate hospital after suffering gunshot wounds.

At age thirty-two, a wet-behind-the-ears coal miner's son from a remote island off the east coast of Canada, I couldn't quite believe that my journey to LA (for a residency program in emergency medicine) had landed me on the set of a popular television series. I did my best to wrestle the stories back to reality. More than once, I had to browbeat the writers into abandoning the notion that a heart attack victim could be hale and hearty the day after his near-death experience. In one episode based on real life, a young boy's arm was bloodlessly extracted from a swimming pool drain. In the incident on which the story was based, the unfortunate lad's arm was amputated to save him from a worse fate.

On *Emergency!*, doctors were superhuman. They didn't have affairs. They didn't drink or fall into addiction. Their patients didn't bleed or die. The diagnoses were accurate. The care they delivered was by the book. This all happened by design, of course. Back in the early days of medical shows, the American Medical Association (AMA) exercised a veto[2] over Hollywood scripts. The shows submitted their scripts to the association for approval, which gave them licence to proudly display the AMA's stamp of approval in the credit lines at the end of the show. What did that do for the TV series? Well, back in an era when doctors were bona fide heroes, the AMA endorsement gave their productions credibility. The AMA, for its part, was more interested in projecting a positive image of doctors than portraying a realistic image of the care they delivered. The AMA-*Emergency!* quid pro quo seems strange today, when every doc who appears on shows like *Grey's Anatomy* or *House* is at least as flawed as their real-life counterparts. But it worked for both sides in the 1970s.

Out on the streets of LA, meanwhile, emergency care was still in its error-prone infancy. The legacy ambulance system was cumbersome and time-consuming. Few first responders—dispatched from either the fire departments or the funeral homes—were well trained. Historically, ambulance teams from the city of LA didn't routinely cross into the county or other neighbouring municipalities to treat patients. Ambulance attendants could put on bandages, and most were trained to perform cardiopulmonary resuscitation (CPR), but that was about it.

If a patient at a roadside or in a home was in ventricular fibrillation, in the early months of the EMS program the responding paramedic squad had to drive to a participating hospital, fetch a coronary care nurse, and then take her to the scene where the patient—usually quite dead by then—could be "legally" defibrillated.

By the mid-1970s, *Emergency!* itself was driving public demand for the better emergency healthcare response depicted on the show. It also attracted a new generation of paramedics to a field considered to be, for the first time, sexy. Enrollment in paramedic training courses quadrupled in jig time. In his comprehensive history of emergency medicine in the US, Dr. Brian Zink provides a succinct description of the show's impact:

> Emergency! *did more for recruiting young men and women into EMS than all the government and organized medicine initiatives of those times combined. Almost every EMS provider who came into the field in the early 1970s distinctly remembers* Emergency! *as a positive influence...and for the first time in the world of entertainment, the American public saw an emergency physician who was a credible doctor. They also saw a new standard of care.*[3]

At first, I thought my gig on *Emergency!* was a chump's assignment. As a rookie in the emergency medicine program at LA County Hospital–USC, I was more or less "voluntold" to do the job. Then came the closest thing to a eureka moment I've ever experienced: Bob Cinader's story taught me that celebrities had power. As a skinny Canadian kid fresh out of a residency program in emergency medicine, I was a nobody. In all my time in LA, I never owned a television. But as a guy who was seen hanging around with TV stars, I had a platform, and I was determined to use it. I lobbied for acquiring medical equipment designed for use in the field. I figured out the Byzantine world of LA politics and plunged into the middle of it every day. Most nights, I fell asleep writing an instruction manual for emergency response and pre-hospital care. Mimeographed copies were distributed to paramedics and first responders across the US, the United Kingdom, and Australia. Caregivers were grateful for the guidance provided, regardless of my stick-person drawings. (The training manual is now housed in the Smithsonian.)

From my first year of medical school, my professional mission was to bring the pioneering field of emergency medicine into the twentieth century. In LA, I helped define better standards of care as a script consultant to *Emergency!*. The goal was to close the gap between TV medicine and the emergency care delivered by paramedics and other healthcare professionals in big, beautiful LA. Good that my patients were surviving on the screens. Better still if more lived to see another day on the streets.

CHAPTER 1

CHILDHOOD IN A COAL-MINING TOWN: SEVERED FINGERS AND SINGED REPORT CARDS, 1942–1960

DONALD HUGH (HUGHIE) STEWART RARELY VENTURED HOME DURING HIS SHIFTS AS A COAL miner, but one day I looked up from an after-school snack and there he was—my father—standing in the kitchen doorway. He wouldn't be staying long. "Just for my tea," he told my mother, Edith, who always had a strong brew bubbling on the coal stove. Dad said he was on the way to the local hospital to get his thumb "sewed back on." The remnants of his digit were wrapped in a hanky in his pocket. My dad had already lost one finger of his left hand and half a digit off his right. He was determined not to make it three. Fortified with black tea and one of my mom's scones, off he went up the hill to the hospital overlooking the harbour, thumb in pocket. At our little hospital, our beloved family doctor reattached what was left of my father's thumb. And it still worked—more or less.

Like most working men in my hometown of Sydney Mines on Cape Breton Island, part of the Canadian province of Nova Scotia, my dad was a coal miner. Born in 1907, Donald Hughie, as he was called by his mates, went "into the pit" at the age of fourteen. He left school to support his growing family. His father, John Duncan, worked as a blacksmith attending to the horses and the "pit ponies" used underground until machines took over. My dad was lucky—if that's the right word—to get his job in 1922. In 1923, the provincial legislature passed amendments to the Mines Act, prohibiting boys younger than sixteen from working underground. Before then, lads as young as nine went down the mines.[4] They often took jobs as "trappers," opening and shutting the wooden doors or "traps" crucial to the ventilation of the mine shaft. This was dank and dismal work—sitting alone in the dark for twelve hours a day or longer.

For the first twenty-five years of the twentieth century, conditions were brutal in Cape Breton's mines. When my dad began work in the 1920s, the newly formed British Empire Steel Corporation (BESCO) sought to cut back miners' wages by 20 percent, limit the right to strike, and break up the United Mine Workers of America (UMWA). Miners lived in flimsy, cheaply built company houses scarcely better than lean-tos. My father was born and raised in one of them. The dwellings had no insulation from bitter winter weather and no indoor plumbing. By the time the miners paid the company rent for these shacks and settled accounts at the company store, there was precious little to show for their gruelling labour underground. Under these punishing conditions, the company's threat in 1925 to trim wages by 20 percent and cut off credit in the company stores were sparks that set smoldering resistance fires alight. And so, four short years after my dad "went into the pit," conflict erupted in Cape Breton mining communities. Company police fired on strikers, killing a miner—William Davis—and injuring others. Workers responded by raiding company stores and setting fire to company offices.[5]

A tragedy in the Princess Colliery in my hometown showed just how cruel "King Coal" could be. Christmastime was approaching in early December of 1938, so added shifts were slotted in by the company to provide miners an opportunity to pocket extra pay. The "trip" was fully loaded in the early hours of the day when the cable lowering the trollies into the mine slope broke. Fragile wooden cars carrying

250 miners hurtled uncontrollably down the track before crashing at high speed at the bottom of an incline. Some veteran miners, alert to the risk, quickly rolled off the trollies. Others stood up and were decapitated by roof beams. Most miraculously survived. The dead and injured, men and boys, were scattered along the long track snaking under the Atlantic Ocean. Twenty-one were killed; more than sixty were injured—fathers and sons, friends and neighbours, young and old. Twenty children were left fatherless.[6] My dad wasn't on the early shift that day, and he lived to see conditions in the Cape Breton mines improve over his forty-five–plus years underground, thanks to growing union strength, strike action, and hard-won government regulations that better protected miners. The onset of the Second World War in 1939 was also decisive. As the war effort drove greater demand for coal, productivity increased and working conditions improved.

This was all part of my Cape Breton heritage when I was born into a war-weary world on October 11, 1942. Our island juts into the Atlantic like an angry fist. Like islanders everywhere, we are a fiercely independent lot, ready and able to fight our way forward in the world. Our island politics are characterized by a suspicious attitude to the provincial capital of Halifax—on the alien mainland—the city that seems (for many on our island) to attract a disproportionate share of government spending on everything from healthcare to cultural institutions. Cape Breton and mainland Nova Scotia do share close historical ties to the US Northeast—the nearby "Boston states." Traditionally, New England was a destination of choice for Nova Scotia family breadwinners looking for jobs during the Great Depression. In late 1942, though, the war in Europe felt closer to our community than the US border at Maine—as indeed it was. Hamilton Hospital (where I was born) stood above Sydney Harbour, then crowded with convoys of steel- and coal-bearing ships being readied to leave the harbour for Britain. The port of Sydney and its smaller "sister" port across the harbour, North Sydney, became major players in the Battle of the Atlantic raging just beyond the shores of Cape Breton. German U-boats infested the waters of the Cabot Strait close to the harbour, waiting for convoys carrying crucial supplies from the bustling Sydney steel mill and the ramped-up production from the coal mines of Glace Bay, Sydney Mines, and the surrounding towns.[7]

North Sydney was the home port of the only railcar ferry to the British colony of Newfoundland, the *SS Caribou*. On the night of my birth, the German submarine U-69 was heading for Sydney Harbour, waiting beyond the harbour's protective submarine net. On October 14, in the early morning, it fired torpedoes at the *Caribou* as it crossed the Cabot Strait, sinking it within minutes with the loss of 136 souls, including ten infants and children. That tragedy became a part of family lore suggesting I was obliged to live a good life to honour the memory of those children. The loss of the *Caribou* was felt throughout the island; many in North Sydney had close relatives in Newfoundland who had been heading home on the ferry.

Ten or so years after my birth, on the day Dad walked home mid-shift with his severed thumb, I was as inured to the hardships of coal mining as almost everyone else in town. I learned to stay calm in the face of a medical emergency. To panic put people at risk in a mining town. As a boy, I didn't fully understand our stoic credo, but I sure lived by it. Nor did I know that the mining culture on the island spawned some astounding innovations, including its own pioneering medical insurance syst coal towns had an early version of universal healthcare coverage called the "check-off" system. A hospital check-off, which paid for the services of the doctor and of the hospital in town, was deducted from every paycheck of every miner.[8] This early form of medicare served as a model for one of the island's venerated politicians, Allan J. MacEachen (also the son of a miner), who played a key role in the introduction of Canada-wide medical insurance in the 1960s. So, when my dad severed his thumb at the mine when I was a lad, he whistled his way to the hospital without a care about paying any bills to have it reattached.

CHILDHOOD IN A COAL-MINING TOWN, 1942–1960

I was drawn into my father's wider world as a young boy. In the Princess Mine, besides digging coal, he built support structures for tunnels. He also took his skills into the community. Dad would often work on his days off to help mates build a shed in a backyard or do some home repairs. He was never paid for this. He knew his mates would pitch in when he needed their help. By the time I was six or seven, I would go with my father to "help" on projects. I'd been equipped with a smaller version of his tool kit, minus anything that was sharp or dangerous to life or limb.

I was an early innovator when it came to building things, another forerunner of a medical career in which I worked to improve various medical devices. My friends and I loved to roam the town's wooded areas where we built secret forts. In the forests we re-enacted the historic British-French struggles for North America played out at the nearby French Fortress of Louisbourg. After finding an "abandoned" bicycle pump I decided to build our own version of an eighteenth-century cannon. We assembled our weapon from the remnants of an old bicycle, the bike pump, a flashlight battery, some tape, and a few pieces of scrap lumber. We removed the piston from the bike pump, screwed off the bottom, and drilled a small hole for the wick of a firecracker to poke through the chamber from inside the pump. We then mounted the pump's steel pipe cylinder on a T-shaped platform built of two-by-fours. Next, we connected the whole contraption to two tire-less bicycle wheels. All we needed was a "D" size flashlight battery stuffed down the pump's cylinder with a broom handle, and all was ready.

When we lit the firecracker fuse—bang—the battery flew out of sight. Birds scattered after the detonation and every eight-year-old in our gang knew we were now rulers of our forest kingdom. Alas, if I fancied myself king, my reign was to be short-lived. My cannon was confiscated and "repurposed" by my father who had heard the cannon's blast, came to investigate, and warned me of the dangers of simulated warfare. My dreams of conquest fell as certainly as had Fortress Louisbourg.[9]

Just as my dad introduced me to carpentry, he gave me an opportunity to practice medicine (or play at it) at an early age. By the time I was born, Donald Hughie was a member of the elite core of draegermen. In the collieries of the island, draegermen were trained in the art and science of mine rescue techniques, first aid, and disaster management. Draeger crews were charged with rescuing trapped or injured workers, fighting fires, shoring up collapsed walls or roofs, repairing damaged lines and equipment, and administering immediate medical care to the injured. This last task interested me from an early age. I would examine every bit of first aid equipment my dad had when he would bring home his "kit" to check the supplies and ensure it was ready to go at a moment's notice. Dad made up a kit for me (less anything sharp or potentially toxic), complete with a red cross, and I was all set for medical adventures. Although I was too young to get a spot on our baseball team, I became the "first aid guy"—equipped with a kit "just like in the pit." Both the kit and I saw little action during the baseball season; I treated one stubbed toe suffered by an outfielder who, I think, was more intent on sitting out the game than playing ball.

When I was not roaming the woods or treating malingering ball players, my life was governed mostly by the demands of school and church. My sister, Donalda, five years my elder, and I were deeply involved in the programs of St. Andrew's Presbyterian Church, and Calvinist doctrine permeated many aspects of our everyday life. The "Christian Sabbath," Sunday, was strictly observed. This meant attending not only a morning worship service but, for my sister and me, Sunday school in the afternoon and family evening service at 7:00 P.M., followed by a youth group meeting. Sunday, often referred to simply as "the Sabbath" mirrored the Jewish holy day as far as prohibitions and restrictions were concerned. Play, fun, music—all were frowned upon, if not forbidden. Housekeeping activities were limited to meal preparation. The cruellest edict for us kids banned swimming in the harbour on Sundays during our short, sweet, warm summer. We were envious of the Catholics kids, who were apparently immune to the fire and brimstone expected to befall those of us who dared to take a Sabbath dip in the harbour—or, God forbid, ride a bike.

Despite religious differences, most people on our island got along well enough—except when it came to hockey. My dad was a rabid fan of our unofficial national sport. We all followed the National Hockey League, but the games that generated the most excitement were local. We had our own team on the north side of Sydney Harbour, ready to fight—literally—for dominance over the teams from Glace Bay, Sydney, New Waterford, and other communities from "cross the harbour." Local hockey teams fought hard for coveted trophies. As did the fans! My dad took me to the games at the Northside Community Forum, but we seldom, if ever, *sat* during the games. Rather, my father positioned us in the "standing-room-only" section, atop the bleachers and near an exit.

I understood why after attending one of my first Saturday night games. While players battled it out on the ice, and sometimes in the penalty box, tension rose in the stands. Indeed, it was not unusual for the worst donnybrooks to take place among the fans. After the siren sounded to end one memorably spirited match, fans poured onto the ice as players retreated to the safety of the dressing rooms. The ice surface was packed with people duking it out. Soon the town's entire police force appeared (both of them), reinforced by the mining company's constabulary, and they put into high gear their version of crowd control. Suddenly and without fanfare, "God Save the King" blared from a scratchy recording over the loudspeaker. Many of the combatants ceased fighting to stand at attention. These stalwarts were rewarded for their misplaced patriotism by being herded through the maintenance doors of the forum into an ancient bus reserved for such occasions. As the story was later told, it took three or four reruns of the royal anthem to contain the mayhem. We didn't wait to count. Dad and I were out of there at the first sign of trouble.

Some of the brawlers, in preparation for the game, had no doubt taken a snort or two of the demon rum. But the strictest of social prohibitions in our happy home fell on the use, at any time or for any occasion, of alcohol. To say our family was teetotal would be an understatement. My grandmother on Mom's side, Charlotte, was a leader in the local branch of the Women's Christian Temperance Union (WCTU), which was very active in Nova Scotia in the first half of the twentieth century. Drinking alcohol simply had no place in our lives. Smoking was equally verboten. Our town had one tavern, located on the main street close to the Salvation Army Citadel. The Army's band was often strategically positioned near the pub to convert revellers enjoying a draught or two inside their own shrine, but not near enough for band members to hear the patrons' catcalls and off-key blasphemous renderings of "Abide with Me" or "The Old Rugged Cross." Our family did have one tangential relationship with alcohol. A neighbour up the street was a known bootlegger, and his frequent night visitors always provided us with a sense of excitement at the thought of the felons (and sinners) in our midst. We always enjoyed the drama when a police officer, accompanied by some helpers, would reluctantly—and oddly enough, unsuccessfully—raid the place.

Fortunately, music, not booze, was the common thread uniting the people of our community. I was gifted with a good singing voice, as was my sister, and as music was one of the few extracurricular programs in our school system, we grabbed the chance to take it up. We never had a keyboard instrument in our home, but the church had several, including a huge pipe organ with an array of levers, pedals, and stops that boggled my preteen mind. So, with a little help from the Presbyterian minister, Doug Wilson, I was able to gain access to the church pianos and organs. It was often assumed I was particularly devout. In truth, I frequented church more to play, not to pray.

Mind you, I would have resorted to prayer to avoid a close relationship with Miss Beatrice Shinners, out town's elite music teacher. Everyone called her "Beat" but never to her face. Unabashedly English in every respect, she carried her rather ample presence around town with a flare the royal family would have envied. In fact, to me she looked exactly like Queen Victoria—plump, round of face, greying hair tightly coiled into a bun atop her head. Her steely and all-seeing eyes squinted through small pince-nez spectacles clipped firmly to her nose. High Anglican to the core, she lived in a huge Victorian house with her brother, Johnny. (Johnny was thought to be "not quite right" which, in our small town, could cover a multitude of eccentricities.) Apparently, the suspicion that I was "musically gifted" leaked into the public domain. She was determined I would become her star pupil and enhance the prestige of her annual "Miss Shinners's Spring Musicale"—held, of course, in the Church of England's decaying hall. I had as much intention of becoming the star of that tea-and-crumpet parade as I did of subjecting myself to Miss Shinners's weekly drills and discipline. My mom didn't press the issue with me at first but began to waver after a "royal visit" from the piano teacher herself. She eventually agreed to put me at Beat's mercy, most likely to rid herself of Miss Shinners's incessant phone calls.

I showed up at Miss Shinners's house all spit-'n'-polish, feeling awkward and resentful that my own mother had caved in the face of bullying, however dressed-up and Anglican. I had the royal carpet laid out—treats and all—with Johnny lurking in the background and peeking menacingly from behind overstuffed chairs and dust-laden ancient furniture. I was ushered with much ceremony into the music room in which Miss Beat worked her magic. It was a small addition to the dining room, with a frosted glass door and a huge piano that took up most of the room. Miss Shinners's bulk occupied the rest. The "lesson" was mercifully short, consisting of my attempts to copy Miss Beat's demonstrations of scales and fingering exercises. While I practised, I was nervously aware of Johnny prowling around the door and fidgeting with the doorknob. Mercifully, the time came for me to exit, but as I planned a hasty retreat, the doorknob came off in Miss Shinners's hand—to the obvious delight of Johnny, who was chuckling on the other side of the door. No number of threats, entreaties, or Biblical verses solved our problem; Johnny just kept on giggling.

Not to be outdone, Miss Shinners decided the window offered the most practical solution. Boosting me up, she instructed me to clamber through the open window, run around to the front door of the house and rescue her. At first, I did as I was told—I just wanted to get out of there. My exuberance was short-lived though, when I realized her prize rose bushes were immediately beneath the window. In full bloom, the roses were surrounded by a host of fully ripe thorns. As for *her* rescue, she would have to see to that herself. I was *not* going back into *that* house of horrors—a Victorian hulk that was surely haunted in the fervid imaginations of my gang of friends. I lit out for home, looking as if I had been through a major war—scratched, with clothes soiled and pungent from recently applied rosebush fertilizer. My mother assumed I had skipped my lesson with Miss Shinners and snuck off with my mates to the local woods rather than pursue my destiny as a musician. In a later—and last—conversation with my mum, Miss Shinners gushed over the great promise I displayed during what she was convinced was a prologue to my musical fame. It was no pro-logue—it was my merciful finale with her!

My dad did launch me on another musical adventure, however. He was a disciple of the great Highland bagpipe, a gift, so the legend goes, of ancient Celtic deities. Pipe music on the island was revered, especially after the founding of a Gaelic college that taught "the pipes" as well as the Gaelic language, Scottish fiddle music, arts, and crafts.

In its early days in the late 1930s, the college ran courses only in the summer, and the tuition was well beyond the reach of a miner's family. To correct this deficit, the college established "winter schools" throughout Cape Breton that offered classes in Highland piping and drumming. The word "winter" on the poster first caught my eye and my interest. I should have taken it as a warning. These gatherings were often held in long-neglected buildings, some old Orange Lodges or Temperance Union gathering places, others in dilapidated church halls. All were either unheated or weakly warmed by an assortment of primitive stoves, with scant provision for fuel save for the furniture we occasionally burned to stave off hypothermia. To survive the lessons, one had to be equipped with mitts or gloves quickly donned between pipe tunes to ensure fingers were not frostbitten but remained supple enough to produce a semblance of musical notes on the practice "chanter." I advanced as an aspiring piper, frostbite notwithstanding, but the classes ended before I graduated to the actual instrument.

No worries; my dad had other plans. He found a "private tutor." John Alex MacNeil, known by most as "John Alex the Piper" was thought to be one of the few pipers who had survived "the War," (meaning the First World War) in which these unfortunate souls were expected to march "over the top" with the first wave of troops. This often-fatal musical charge was designed to spur the troops on to victory, as well as to scare the enemy into immediate retreat or surrender. In John Alex's telling of it, pipers would lead the charge into no man's land, kilts wafting in the wind, taking pride in being known by German soldiers as "the women from hell." John Alex was honoured more for surviving the war than for his marksmanship or, certainly, his piping skills. No matter, Dad had done some carpentry work for John Alex, and it was payback time.

The only time available for us to head over to Sydney, where John Alex lived, was on Saturday mornings because Dad had to borrow a car from a friend. At that time, a half-hour journey around the harbour to Sydney was considered a grand adventure. And so it was for me, my excitement heightened by the thought I would be taking lessons from a war hero. Only one problem faced us: my tutor was a frequent fixture at a local watering hole along the waterfront of Sydney—even early in the mornings. The pub was known to skirt government rules and was under the watchful, though "unofficial," prying eyes of the Women's Christian Temperance Union. Being of Calvinist persuasion, it would be unheard of for either my dad or me to enter the premises, even to save a lost soul who happened to be a master of the Highland bagpipe. Still, I was delegated to enter the pub and retrieve my "hero." This was no errand for the faint of heart. By this time, mid-morning, John Alex was well fortified from playing requested tunes in exchange for draughts of ale. I somehow extracted him from the pub; he joined me and my dad in the car to drive to his house where the lesson was to take place.

The drill there was regimental: He would play a few tunes and I would take his pipes and attempt to repeat at least one of them. Predictably, given the alcohol vapours embedded in the leather bag of the instrument during the morning drink-athon, I never got out more than a tune or two. With more than a few ungodly wails issuing from the offended instrument, I passed out cold on the floor, with a blood alcohol level no doubt equal to my distinguished instructor's. "Ach!" old Alex would say, "he'll be right as rain once he ketches 'is wind. He'll be toughened up in no time, Donald Hughie." I could well have become the youngest member of Alcoholics Anonymous on the island had my lessons continued. They didn't.

"John Alex the Piper" was far from the only denizen of our island known primarily by his nickname.[10] With so many Mac-Somethings in the area, nicknames were used to identify people or families. At one point the mining payrolls of Sydney Mines featured twenty-three "John MacDonalds" and almost as many "John MacNeils." One of our close neighbours, Mr. Alex Saddler, was a good friend, but I was well into my teen years before I realized his "real" name was Alex MacDonald. His father had been a saddler and kept horses; Alex never did, but the name followed him. The naming traditions within the coal mining culture of the island have been the focus of scholarly work both in Cape Breton and beyond. Nicknames could reflect the miner's birthplace or where he might currently live—John Caledonia was really John MacDonald who lived in the village of Caledonia, "Sandy Cape North" might live in Cape North, but not necessarily; if for example, his parents moved long ago from there, the name still stuck. Often these names were passed down to later generations. Some nicknames might refer to physical characteristics—the unfortunate "Donnie Clock" had been born with Erb's palsy, a birth injury that leaves one arm shorter than the other. Nicknames were even used in the official papers of the mining bureaucracy. "Neil Bottom" worked at the bottom of the mine shaft. Alex Cage operated the elevator down the shaft. "Horse Shit Dan" cared for the ponies. Nicknames applied not only to the miners but often carried over to wives or families; "Kate Black Angus" was the wife of Angus MacDonald, who often would not shower in the facilities on the mine surface but would head home to wash up. It was not unknown to find these names used on formal and legal documents, and sometimes on tombstones.

I'm not sure whether the tag "John Alex the Piper" followed him to his gravesite, but I do know he was the first and last private tutor I endured as a youth growing up in Sydney Mines. Neither he nor those cold community halls could extinguish my lifelong love of music— which was still alive and well later in my life when I incorporated music and the arts into the curriculum at the Dalhousie Medical School. Of course, I developed other interests as I grew into my teen years. Excelling in school (and everything else) was a goal born of an unbridled competitive spirit. My parents expected me to "do good" in school. The measure of success was top marks on tests or exams. I usually did well, driven in part by my competition with my friend and classmate, Anita MacDowell. In one instance, when I placed second to her in my class, I stormed home from school and promptly threw my report card into the kitchen stove. My exasperated mother retrieved it and—waving the singed card in front of me—followed up with a lecture about humility, the need to share in others' successes, and the perils of getting "too big for your britches." At my mom's insistence, I paid an immediate visit to Anita and congratulated her. I *did* try to be sincere; and while my attempt at reconciliation did little to lighten my dark mood, my mom certainly got her point across.

School was one thing—sports another. Curling, the ancient Scottish version of chess on ice, was a beloved game in our area. I threw myself into the sport—so much so that by grade 11 I was made "skip," or captain, of our team for the province-wide playoffs in Sydney. But the week before we headed around the harbour, the coach of the team felt that one of my best buds, Jimmy Caldwell—in grade 9, two grades below me—should replace me as skip. At that news I was ready to throw in the broom. My mother bore the brunt of my daily whining and, as usual, she did a pretty good job of convincing me to concentrate on the fact that I was on a winning team. It turned out Jimmy did well after replacing me as skip, and we led the playoffs for a day or two. We managed to beat the big-city team from Queen Elizabeth High School in Halifax, an upset of such epic proportions the local press christened us "the Cinderella team." That brief moment of glory soothed my bruised ego. (Jimmy and I were to remain close friends even beyond our graduating year from Sydney Mines High School, until his tragic death in a car accident about a year later.)

It was only when I later looked back at my years in Sydney Mines that I realized how fortunate Donalda and I were in our home life. Our family unit sailed ahead on an even keel—no sea-storms or rogue waves put us off course. Certainly, our adherence to the basic tenets of Calvinist/Presbyterian belief systems favoured humility, peace, hard work, and security, and both my parents seemed to lead by example.

Rudeness was not tolerated, and I never witnessed my parents exchange words in anger. They also took leadership roles in the community, Dad as a Scout leader, Mom as a member of women's clubs and charities that reached out to people confined to their homes by ill health. More than anyone I knew growing up, my mother would reach out across the unspoken religious, racial, economic, and political boundaries that divided our community. Heck, she even allowed a devout Anglican—who thought me a musical prodigy—to teach me piano. And she always made sandwiches and baked goods for the Indigenous (Mi'kmaw) people who (once or twice a year) travelled door-to-door selling hand-woven baskets. Mom would tell me, time and time again, that the Mi'kmaw women worked hard to sell their beautiful handcrafts, travelling all day with heavy loads on their backs. If I later took even a quarter of her compassion and her openness into my medical practice, my patients benefitted from her example.

My most prominent influence outside my family during my teenage years was the minister, Doug Wilson, who presided at St. Andrew's from 1954 to 1962. I relied on "Reverend Doug" for advice about any major decisions, and he served as a trustworthy sounding board for a variety of adolescent growing pains. One of his helpers in his work with young people in the town was Lawrence Stewart, a close friend and distant relative about nine years my elder. Lawrence left school in grade 10 or so and worked in our local Co-op, the main general store on Main Street. He became deeply involved in Mr. Wilson's programs for young people and soon began to show a real interest in going back to school—perhaps to follow in the reverend's footsteps. (Lawrence's life and mine were destined to intertwine in the most tragic of ways, as you'll read in the next chapter.)

Oddly enough, given their Calvinist quirks, neither of our parents was legalistic or strict about "rules." In fact, rules and even laws were judged in our mining society as sometimes optional, depending largely on the urgency of a situation in which they might be broken or the likelihood of being caught. The decisive factor as to whether laws or rules should be obeyed was whether someone was harmed or at risk if such were at the most clearly broken or at the least slightly bent. This applied always to fishing licences or permits to do this or that—and particularly to motor vehicles. My dad figured there was no compelling reason on God's green earth why his son shouldn't be allowed to drive an old Oldsmobile after he passed his fourteenth birthday—two years before I could legally obtain a licence. (Later in life, in my rural Cape Breton medical practice, I would have to take some licence myself to provide proper care not only as a trained doc but as an untrained dentist, coroner, undertaker, and veterinarian.)

Back in my early teens, my access to a car widened my social circle significantly. I was set free with the family car, based largely on the fact that Dad trusted me. (Even then I suspected my popularity wasn't due to my sparkling personality). Soon enough, our circle of chums, girls and boys, would venture around the harbour to the "South side"—Sydney and its suburbs, where the "uppity" people lived. Thinking back, they weren't that wealthy, but they were richer and thought themselves more sophisticated than us kids from the "North side." My trips to the Sydney area also took me on my first journey into heartbreak. Mary was her name, her surname lost to memory and to history. But she seemed eager to take up with a fourteen-year-old (with a car), even one from "the Mines." Besides, there was a special dance coming up at our school—the event of the year—and it would have enhanced my social standing should I show up in a car with a Sydney girl on my arm. Wow! But disaster slowly sunk my ship of hope as soon as several of Mary's friends got legal drivers' licences and I was left without a hope of romance and adventure 'round the harbour. Life can be cruel.

In the mid-1950s, Donalda left for Ontario to pursue a career in meteorology in the Canadian Forces. By that time, I had begun to prepare for high school. The loss of my sister to "Upper Canada" was difficult for my parents. By the time she left, we had moved to another house, a small bungalow situated in a neighbour's backyard. I was quite happy about it—I had my own room, and the house was closer to the high school. I welcomed the variety of "stuff" I could get involved in at high school, including the curling and basketball teams. Our high school had neither a lab nor a gym of any kind, so our basketball practice was held in the gym of a new high school in the neighbouring town of North Sydney. Lab work was limited to reading about experiments and understanding how things *should* work out, without actually *doing* them. Most of the teachers were well along in their careers and focussed largely on the humanities. Latin was mandatory, with lessons starting in grade 6 or 7. Our principal, Mrs. Adeline Purves, a dedicated and experienced teacher, lived and breathed Latin and English literature. It was no accident, then, that I came out of high school steeped in the humanities but with a gnawing curiosity about science. By June of 1960, when I graduated, I was ready to step out into a wider world by leaving home for university—and into a new decade and a new era to boot.

CHAPTER 2

LOVE, LOSS, AND ONE GIANT EXPLOSION, 1960–1965

I HAD HOPED TO ARRIVE AT ACADIA UNIVERSITY AS A SOLO ROMANTIC FIGURE STEPPING OFF the train with a dusty old duffel bag in hand—like the protagonist in a James Dean movie or a silent soldier just returned from the wars. Alas, I wasn't fated to travel alone on the journey toward my future in the small university town of Wolfville, Nova Scotia. I was a miner's son from a small town, leaving for university. This was an event, and I was lucky the whole town didn't see me off. As it turned out, Mom and Dad insisted on coming with me on the journey, along with two sets of neighbours in two other cars. Together, our entourage had packed enough food to feed half the campus. All the farewell weeping and wailing that should have happened in Sydney Mines would be displayed on the Acadia campus instead—in full view of classmates and (horrors) "upper classmen." (This latter species salivated at any excuse to make "freshman" initiation rituals particularly excoriating.) If I had planned to look cool—though "hip" would probably have been the right word in 1960—it sure didn't work out that way.

I was drawn to Acadia University in Wolfville by its small-town setting, religious affiliation with the Baptist church, and the beauty of the Annapolis Valley. Acadia was also Doug Wilson's old school. The charismatic clergyman had nudged me toward his alma mater, where he had served as managing editor of the student newspaper, treasurer of the students' union, and class president for all four years of his degree. He was right; Acadia was a good fit for me. With around nine hundred students, the university was small enough to provide a soft landing for a seventeen-year-old kid from Sydney Mines, and large enough to be academically sound. Doug also left behind big shoes to fill at the university, and I avoided trying to walk in them. I was happy to traipse about in my own size tens and see where they would take me. Happily, just before leaving my hometown I found out my cousin Lawrence Stewart had graduated from high school with honours. He too was coming to Acadia to do a BA before heading off to theological college in Montréal. I would have a friend on campus.

Lawrence helped me survive it all—and to endure my student digs on campus. I was assigned to accommodations in the basement of War Memorial House, a residence better known as Barrax. The suite featured two bedrooms and housed three students. I shared the bigger room with a fellow first-year student I can barely remember. My other roommate—the sole occupant of what could have been a monk's cell or an old broom closet—became a lifelong friend. Walter Borden, an African Nova Scotian, was himself a bit monkish. He was unique—a poet and an aesthete. He only went to classes he liked—mostly English and drama. He stayed in his room reading books the rest of us never heard of. I wouldn't doubt that the school (in the royalist territory of Kings County) had stashed him in the most obscure part of the campus. And as a Black scholar in the middle of an (almost) all-white school of jocks, he was shunned by many students.

Walter and I were both born in 1942. We both grew up in small towns in Nova Scotia—New Glasgow, in Walter's case. We both came from areas with strong historic links to the coal-mining industry. Both of us would later become nationally recognized—me in medicine, Walter in the arts. Both of us would be named to the Order of Canada. Our backgrounds united us, to some degree, but I knew even then that

I didn't have to endure his lot in life. Walt, who would mature into an irrepressibly animated man, retreated into his shell at Acadia. He would only go to the dining hall toward the end of mealtimes—after almost everyone else had left. I tried to meet up with him to enjoy his company at meals, but I also wanted to include him with my other friends. Having Walt there inevitably made even the dining hall food more palatable. I still recall the conversation of our fellow students coming to an abrupt halt when Walter and I walked into a room together. They were talking about him, and he knew it.

Walter Borden would become an accomplished actor, poet, playwright, and ardent human rights activist. But the budding human rights advocate only occasionally flowered into his full glory at Acadia. Occasionally, Walter would grow frustrated when people expressed surprise that he spoke in a down-home accent at a time when Nova Scotia universities were more likely to educate Africans than African Nova Scotians. "I'm from New Glasgow, not Mozambique," the small-framed Borden would declaim to his startled interlocuters in his booming voice—a thespian's instrument destined for the stage. In his occasional exuberant moods, the monkish reader would proclaim his destiny and break into his falsetto parody of the Reverend Mother's "Climb Every Mountain" from the then-popular Broadway musical hit *The Sound of Music*. And I would collapse in laughter. I was crestfallen to discover, in the fall of 1961, that Walter was not returning to Acadia for a second year of studies. Decades later, we would meet again by chance in a theatre in Halifax, he on one side of the curtain, I on the other.

At Acadia, I attempted to become a player of a different kind—not as an actor but as a card shark. The stereotypical undergraduate experience wasn't for me. Calvinism aside, I never understood the attraction of getting sloshed out of my mind on booze and lying around semi-comatose in the aftermath of a binge. But as a kid from Cape Breton, I was supposed to excel at two things—drinking and playing cards—so I decided to forego the former and take up the latter. To comic effect, as it turned out. I had a major disadvantage—being steeped in the Calvinist aversion to playing cards, I knew nothing about such wickedness—not even the names of the cards, so I would hang around watching my fellow students play "hearts" until I thought I half understood the game and the symbols on the cards. Seemed easy—hearts look like hearts, diamonds like diamonds. My career as a card shark exploded during my very first game when I triumphantly threw down what I thought was the winning card and announced, "the six of CLOVERS." The laughter still haunts.

Despite my missteps, I soaked up everything in Wolfville and on the campus. Before I went there, I had never heard a symphony or watched a professional stage play—or played a game of cards. It was all new to me. I went to lectures delivered in halls accommodating up to 150 other students, at what could have been Harvard or Cambridge. I loved studying, and let curiosity guide my course selection. I certainly didn't want to study *only* what I already knew, so I took Latin, Greek, French and medieval French philosophy. In the process, I became fairly fluent in French.

My fervent interest in the language was linked to the arrival of a new troupe of female students housed off campus in a once-elegant inn, Blomidon House, on the edge of town. Two of these young women were to become close friends. Karen MacDonald was a warm and poised young woman who grew up across Sydney Harbour from my hometown. She was one of the "Blomidon girls" who had an aura of mystery because they lived off campus on the edge of town. They travelled to and from Acadia on an antiquated bus soon dubbed "the Iron Maiden." Karen and I talked mostly about our island home, but I also benefitted from her view of Acadia life and her reviews of the current campus buzz. A deep friendship took root, with my hopes it would blossom into something intimate and long-lasting.

I enjoyed an even closer relationship with Karen's good friend, Brita Stolz, a fellow student in several small French classes. Born in Germany, she had also lived in France. She was also a stunning beauty on the little campus in Wolfville. She didn't show a trace of arrogance despite her obvious gifts and sophistication—or perhaps because of them. I became a smitten eighteen-year-old. But the competition for her approval was fierce. Members of the football team clamoured for her attention, and I would volunteer my opinions of her hapless suitors whether she asked for it or not. (Can't say I gave any of them a favourable review. Besides, I hated football. I thought it was a horrible thing to kick people around like that.) But I confess I was frustrated by the self-imposed limitations of my friendship with Brita. We shared our secrets and genuinely enjoyed each other's friendship. But I didn't want to be her guardian or her confidante; I wanted more. Alas, it was not to be.

Our backgrounds—I was a kid from a coal town, she was an Old World sophisticate—were anything but similar. Still, we developed a close friendship. I could easily confide in her about my nascent plans to become a doctor, and almost anything else. She was a visual artist in every way and could sculpt a friendship as deftly as she painted a portrait or landscape. My appreciation for her art paid a long-term dividend; it helped cement the bond that drew us back together long after we left Acadia. But both she and Karen showed me that you could have a relationship with women that wasn't just about hormones. Though life would take Karen, Brita, and me in different directions, our bonds held fast; and just as with Walter Borden, I would reunite and reconnect with them decades after we had first met at Acadia.

One of the great advantages of Acadia was the close relationship students could cultivate with professors and staff at the university. Because my French and more advanced classes were small, relationships with professors were often warm, friendly, and personal. Toward the end of my arts degree, I was asked by one of my French professors to become her assistant, a job that entailed correcting undergraduate assignments and, in my case, helping to run the language laboratory. This latter role was nearly my undoing, since my professor, whom I got to know well, suffered from a serious mental illness. I spent many hours accompanying her to hospitals or rescuing some poor freshman who was the victim of her fits of psychotic rage. My relationship with her provided an early, utterly untutored, lesson in managing patient relationships.

My most important mentors during my latter years at Acadia— just as I was finishing my arts degree—were two biologists: the dean of science, Chalmers Smith, and his wife, Ada Smith. I sought their advice because I gradually realized I was leaning toward medical school and would need a science degree to qualify. They invited me to tea at their home atop the hill overlooking the campus. Both encouraged me to consider transferring to science after my BA degree, but Professor Smith suggested I consider whether I was the "medical type," which, in his opinion, meant being able to adopt a dispassionate, "uninvolved" view of patients and their needs. This advice confused me and, after several days of replaying our conversation in my mind, distressed me. I soon was back having yet another tea at the Smiths. I told him frankly that my concept of what a physician requires was the opposite of what he cautioned me against. Didn't caring for patients *require* that a physician get "involved"—appropriately—in their care, and that *empathy* was essential? His smile and a nodding acknowledgement from Mrs. Smith gave me a sense not of having "won" the point, but rather that I had answered any lingering doubts they might have had. My decision was made then and there: I would go to medical school. I enrolled in the science faculty for the fall semester in 1963 and spent two more years at Acadia.

✱

It turned out the 1963–64 academic year was formative in a way I could never have anticipated. As the years passed, I had become closer and closer to my cousin Lawrence when I hitched rides with him on the weekends in his yellow Volkswagen Beetle and we talked about life, love, studying, and our futures. He'd drive as far as his parish church in Pictou (three hours away), and I'd hitchhike from there to Sydney Mines to visit my folks. Our chatter flowed easily—and loudly. (We had to tax our vocal cords just to be heard above the roar emitting from the VW exhaust system.) As the son of a man who tinkered with cars endlessly and could fix anything, I was handy enough myself to be irritated by the unmuffled racket the VW made. It didn't seem to bother Lawrence, who treated the interior of the car as a living space. The back seat was piled high with laundry, which Lawrence took home to wash on weekends, and with blankets for protection against Nova Scotia's unpredictable winter weather—sunshine one moment, a blizzard the next. Winter conditions sometimes brought traffic to a standstill until a snowplow happened by. Lawrence would sometimes curl up somewhere alongside the winding road through the Rodden Hills en route to Pictou and catch a few winks. He also kept a stash of high caloric "comfort food" and Coke in the car to keep him awake. We made good use of the time—parsing Greek verbs or reading Greek passages assigned by our professor. Sometimes, I'd correct his Greek— languages came more easily to me. During one of our trips I told him about my determination to study medicine. When he told me to think about it for a while, I could hear the disappointment in his voice. He was still clinging to the hope I would follow him into the Church, but I had rejected that option years previously, and not only because of my discussions with Doug Wilson. Truth was, by the time I left home, I was seriously questioning my faith in a rigid religious doctrine that raised more questions than it answered.

While Lawrence was studying theology at Acadia, his life seemed to be moving forward at breakneck speed. Just before Christmas holidays in 1963, Lawrence surprised us all by announcing he had met a girl in Pictou County and intended to marry her. They had set a date—New Year's Eve, 1963—only a few weeks away. Within weeks, a very happy Lawrence was off to Ontario to marry Florence Hood, who was also closely tied to the Presbyterian faith. Lawrence and Florence enjoyed a short honeymoon before returning to Nova Scotia, where my cousin and I met up again at Acadia during the first week of classes in 1964. I made him promise that I could hitch a ride with him the next Friday to Pictou, where I would meet his bride before continuing to Cape Breton. Lawrence gave me marching orders to meet him precisely at 3:00 P.M. on January 17, 1964, to head out of town. He had good reasons to depart on time: he was anxious to meet Florence, of course, but in addition, the weather had been worthy of the Russian steppes that week. A major snowstorm days before the planned trip had left the roads all but impassable. Better to travel in the daylight as much as possible, then. I prepared for the getaway by packing my small knapsack for the weekend, then headed to a class in a biology lab. As luck would have it, I was unable to sneak out early as we were dissecting cats, with our professor paying far too much attention to our somewhat hurried dissection. After I was finally set free, I sprinted for my rendezvous with Lawrence, only to see his yellow VW pull away while I slipped and slid on the icy ground. He didn't spot me in the rear-view mirror, and I was left stranded as the Bug disappeared in a puff of snow.

Later that evening, a call from the Royal Canadian Mounted Police was routed to my residence number from the main Acadia switchboard. It sounded official. I answered in yes-sirs and no-sirs to a constable who said some Mounties were heading over to campus to see me. What did I do? I didn't have a car, so it couldn't be some outstanding ticket; I hadn't been in a major brawl—then or ever. The sombre look on the faces of the two officers who arrived at the residence shortly thereafter should have alerted me to something really, really bad.

My recollection of what was said is half-lost in a fog of disjointed memories.

"We're so sorry to tell you…"

"Would you like to use our phone to call your home?"

"Do you need any help with packing…?"

"We have a car waiting to drive you home to the island."

Slowly things fell into place…bits and pieces of their recounting of what had happened. "Transport truck…slid over the centre line… fell on top of Mr. Stewart's Volkswagen…he didn't suffer…killed instantly…his front-seat passenger in hospital, in serious condition… may not make it."

What? What front-seat passenger? That was *my* seat; *I* should have been there. (As it turned out, this was not to be my last near-brush with death—but more on that later.) I was always there with Lawrence driving. Why wasn't I there? I wasn't terribly coherent, but I recalled that we had intended to pick up one of our classmates who needed a ride toward his home in Moncton, New Brunswick. He was now hanging on to life and not expected to survive.

The rest of the week—and to some extent, the term—was a blur. I did finally meet his wife of seventeen days, Florence, as we stood together watching a flower-draped casket being lowered into the snow-covered rocky ground of his Cape Breton home. (I never was to see her again.) I recall little or nothing of that day, only that I faced going back to familiar surroundings at Acadia—his familiar surroundings. I concentrated on the task I had been asked to carry out—packing up all of Lawrence's things to bring home the next weekend to his parents. I still was in a fog, but I did it.

I tried my best to keep up my usual pace afterward, but I remained trapped in a sort of limbo. Studying seemed beyond my reach, as was going to class and even eating. Nothing interested me; nothing seemed to matter. I learned that I could hide most of this, except for missing classes. By then I was heavy into laboratory work and research in biology dissection as well as biochemistry. Most labs required partners, and to miss even one was not only academically risky but unfair to a partner. But even knowing that didn't seem to stir me into action. It was only with the support of a gang of my close Acadia buddies that I began to emerge from the shadows. I slowly got back on the academic track and was able, with the help of lab partners and very understanding professors, to catch up academically and generally feel on my feet again. At this point, I came to rely on Brita.

It was because of Brita, Karen, and other friends, that I screwed up enough courage to knock on the door of the university physician, Dr. Sutherland, whom I knew only slightly. It was hard for me to admit I needed help. Dr. Sutherland was a good listener, and after several sessions I began to realize how deeply affected I was by Lawrence's death. I couldn't answer the big questions that were gnawing at me—why can't I just pick myself up, dust off, and get on with life? But it wasn't that simple. The rigid and rather narrow confines of my pre-packaged Calvinist thinking couldn't take the strain of what had happened, and I needed a reset. (It was only in looking back, years later, that I realized I had the classic signs of clinical depression.)

An old-fashioned remedy—intense activity—seemed to help in restoring me to health. At the urging of friends, I plunged into a campaign to run for president of the Acadia students' union for the 1964–65 academic year. This was during an era of intense student activism on North American campuses. It had started back in 1960–61, my first year at Acadia. While Walter Borden was keeping a sort of lonely vigil as a rare Black student in a residence at Acadia, thousands of American college students were joining the Student Nonviolent Coordinating Committee and the Freedom Riders. In the summer of 1961, hundreds of young people from US campuses travelled to the deep south to fight for civil rights—and some died in the effort. By my final year on campus, protests against the Vietnam War were just starting to heat up. At Acadia, it was as if the outside world didn't exist. So much so that I positioned my campaign as a protest against student apathy, which seemed more evident to me when other candidates withdrew their intention to offer for president after I submitted mine. But I wasn't about to rely on winning an election by default. At a university where voter turnout for student elections rarely hit 55 percent, I published an editorial in the *Athenaeum,* the student newspaper, proposing a referendum on whether or not I should accept the presidency. As I explained,

> *My reasons for doing this are twofold: one, so that you may, after all, elect a president, and two, if elected by a majority of students, then I shall feel that I enjoy your support and will have confidence to carry the heavy responsibility of serving you. There is yet another reason. In the past we [students] at Acadia have been accused of apathy. This is our chance to prove ourselves worthy of a strong student government by supporting the new Union with, at least, our vote on Monday.... And so we do, after all, have a choice.*[11]

This was a bit of an audacious pitch. I was the only candidate in the presidential race, which in itself was enough to induce apathy in the electorate. Still, I worked hard; I gave speeches in every residence common room, narrowly avoiding the 10:00 P.M. curfew in the women's residences—fuelled up no doubt by the thrill of barely escaping the predictable wrath of the House Mother armed with a broom (or worse). The campaign worked—voter turnout on election day was 76 percent. And the YES vote was 97 percent in favour. This lesson in democracy—campaign hard and you might just carry the day—stayed with me; I drew on it decades later when I entered Nova Scotia politics.

I was to learn some other life lessons following my electoral victory in the spring term of 1964. That summer, I ended up in the newly independent country of Algeria, courtesy of an international scholarship that took me to my own personal heart of darkness in Africa. I was travelling as part of what turned out to be a star-studded group of forty-three university students awarded scholarships by the World University Service of Canada to do outreach work. Beverley McLachlin (née Gietz), who later served as the chief justice of the Supreme Court of Canada, was in the group. So were David Dodge, later governor of the Bank of Canada between 2001 and 2008, and Raymond Chrétien, Canada's ambassador to the United States between 1994 and 2000. (I corresponded for years afterward with Beverley Gietz, and only discovered that she was "that Bev"—the distinguished jurist—after she was appointed to Canada's top court in 2000.)

We were assigned to do field work in Algeria after convening in Sainte-Adèle, Quebec, for a one-week orientation. The route to Algiers traced what felt like a romantic route to me, a flight to Paris from Montréal, a journey by train from Gare de Lyon to Marseille, and finally a voyage to the ancient city of Algiers aboard the SS *Kairouan.* Algeria had been administered as a part of France since the early nineteenth century, before a war of independence broke out in 1954. Ten years later, when we arrived there, Algeria was a newly liberated nation. The fighting finally ended in 1962, but the post-colonial nation was anything but stable. We met with Algeria's president, Ahmed Ben Bella, who would be deposed a year later. In addition, the French citizens and other Europeans still living in the country after the war were often blamed for acts of terrorism that continued to occur around the country.

My assignment in Algeria took me to the desert city of Constantine, where I linked up with Bedouin people whose newborns suffered from unusually high rates of tetanus. I soon understood why.

The nomadic peoples of the Sahara had long taken soil and rubbed it into the umbilical cords of babies. The soil itself contained bacilli for tetanus, and high incidences of the disease were an inevitable result. I was to look into the prevalence of tetanus and see what steps could be taken. This was a difficult task because it was a cultural issue. After finishing my field work in Constantine, I travelled to the port city of Annaba (formerly known as Bône), where I would soon learn just how unstable Algeria was. On July 24, 1964, the *Star of Alexandria*, an Egyptian ship loaded with munitions, blew up at dockside.[12] Pieds Noirs, a name given to Europeans born in Africa during the Colonial era, were blamed. They were accused of planting a bomb aboard the vessel, but to this day no one knows for certain who triggered the explosion. We were all staying in an old French army barracks on the outskirts of the city at the time of the explosion, writing up reports on our project work and awaiting flights back to France. I heard the explosion, ran outside, and saw a mushroom-shaped cloud that looked like the one that had arisen over Hiroshima. In no time, shrapnel started to rain down on the tile roofs of the buildings, even though we were about ten kilometres (six miles) away. We all scurried inside and took shelter under the beds. The toll of the disaster was never really known, but at the time, the newspaper *Le Monde* reported there were thought to be more than two hundred deaths.[13] Hundreds more were injured.

After the explosion, I and others from our Canadian group were press-ganged into action by relief officials from the Red Crescent, who put me in charge of a ward at a psychiatric hospital. Almost all the staff seemed to have just run off after the explosion. The windows had blown out and most of the patients had escaped as well. The only ones left were the most severely ill—the ones who had been restrained or locked in rooms and could not escape. The experience piqued my interest in emergency response medicine, but not at a sophisticated level. I provided treatment but I didn't know what I was doing. My main job was to provide food and sustaining care to those who were left. After three days without sleep, I practically wept with joy when I was relieved by members of the Red Crescent and many of the staff, who had returned. I crawled into the nearest corner under a table and slept. After that, I simply left. I wasn't really needed any longer and, as a foreigner with only a smattering of Arabic, I wasn't very useful.

I hitchhiked south, back to Constantine, about 120 kilometres (75 miles) away. I took rides in donkey carts and any other vehicle that would pick me up. (I had an airline return ticket to Paris, leaving from Constantine.) I had just arrived in the city when I was stopped by police and arrested. I was detained at the police station and interrogated, with some difficultly because most of the police there spoke an Arabic dialect or very accented French, of which only a few words seeped through to me. I really don't know why I was under suspicion, except martial law had been declared and I was obviously a foreigner. There seemed to be some suspicion—oddly enough—that I might be linked to the munitions boat explosion. Though the interrogation was not violent, it didn't help one bit that I spoke classical French—in an accent associated with the colonialists who had lost the war but not left the country. After two days in detention, police took me out of my cell in the early morning and marched me to a waiting van. I was too tired to even be alarmed at being hustled into the back of a van in a foreign country headed for who-knows-where. I didn't know what was going on or where I was being taken. I did know it was not a great moment.

To my relief, I was driven to the airport and promptly deported on a flight to Marseille. Paris was my real destination, but I was relieved enough to get back to France, even though it meant sleeping my first night on the ground on the outskirts of the Mediterranean port city. The next day, I hitchhiked from Marseilles to Paris, eventually reuniting with some of my Canadian co-adventurers. During this period, I was writing letters home to my parents that were, quite frankly, a pack of lies. Throughout the years my mother kept the correspondence, in which I said—among other things—that the police "were kind enough to give me a place to stay and drive me to the airport."

✳

Back on campus that fall, I learned too soon that the euphoria of an electoral victory can give way all to quickly to the stark realities of the burdens of office. Within weeks of my swearing in as president of the student union, the student newspaper, the *Athenaeum*, printed an advertisement for the "Aristocrat Tavern" in the nearby town of Kentville. The publication of a liquor ad did not sit well with Acadia's vice-president, Dr. Ronald Stewart Longley, who divested himself of his usual dour but kindly Baptist facade by exploding in a fit of fury. On the same morning the *Athenaeum* was released, I was called to his office "for consultation." There was no consultation; he simply suggested that newspaper staff could not both be part of the university community and ignore the "norms." I took this as a not-so-veiled threat of expulsion of the editorial board, or at least of the editor. My Cape Breton union roots kicked in and I was ready to roll up my sleeves, storm the Baptist barricades, and chance the consequences. But after the initial shock dissipated, I thought the best I could do was at least delay any decisions until I had a chance to meet up with the staff of the *Athenaeum* and plan an approach. I may have mumbled something about taking the situation under advisement— or some such nonsense—simply to get out of the vice-president's office before either blowing my stack or disintegrating into a blubbering mass of tears. I hightailed it out and headed for a class. By the time I got back and sorted myself out as best I could, Dr. Longley had already called a meeting with the *Athenaeum*'s staff and read the riot act. Eventually a deal was worked out under which the editors would publish a "clarification" of the advertisement in the next edition of the newspaper.

Looking back on my Acadia years, I now understand that the university, in some ways, provided me with the safe landing I was looking for when I first enrolled.

Not all that soft, mind you, which turned out to be a good thing for a young man headed toward a career in emergency medicine.

CHAPTER 3

THREE WISE MEN GUIDE ME HOME, 1965–1970

IN 1965, I MOVED FROM WOLFVILLE TO MY OWN VERSION OF MANHATTAN; NOT THE STORIED island of towering skyscrapers but the small provincial capital of Nova Scotia—Halifax. (It felt like a giant metropolis to me.) When people ask me today about my five years at the Dalhousie University Medical School, I usually say the time passed in a blur. Tied to the university and its teaching hospitals, determined to master the curriculum, and not tempted by the port city's legendary waterfront pubs, I rarely roamed beyond the borders of the campus and the surrounding neighbourhoods. My first address was Howe Hall, a student residence that still graces the southwest corner of Coburg Road and LeMarchant Street. The grey stone building showcases its stern architectural elegance to passersby on the street—an elegance utterly unreflective of the bacchanalian milieu I endured inside the residence as a first-year medical student.

I had a private room—but no privacy—on the first floor of Howe Hall. My existence in the aptly nicknamed "jungle" was dominated by first-year undergraduate men (more accurately, boys) away from home for the first time and determined to taste the joys of independence and alcohol. For the most part, their new-found freedom was expressed through loud roughhousing, louder music, and copious consumption of booze. Worse than that, I became the go-to medical counsellor for the whole adolescent herd. I soon learned to retreat to the medical library to study.

My first weeks at medical school proved more instructive, and in one instance more alarming, than residence life. Our class was divided into groups of eight, each assigned its own body in the dissection lab. Studying under the seemingly omnipotent professors in the anatomy department, we soon learned all cadavers were not created equal. Thin ones are preferred, since fat tissue tends to obscure internal anatomy, especially when it comes to tracing the course of a nerve or blood vessel.

In the anatomy lab I experienced the first shock of my medical career. There, on the third table down from our own, lay the remains of a family friend, one of my dad's closest mining pals. I will protect his anonymity, but I can say he was a great guy, always around our house, always ready with a joke. He would often have a "surprise" for me—a sweet of some kind or something he had carved from scraps of wood. After spotting him, I beat a hasty retreat from the lab and went outside into the warm autumn sunshine. I was overwhelmed: this man had given me and the medical school another gift, one that was indeed special. Once I absorbed that fact, I headed back into the lab, gritted my teeth, and picked up my scalpel. I also steered well clear of his cadaver for the rest of the year.

It's no exaggeration to say that a man with my neighbour's background—who gives his body to medical science and education—is a visionary of sorts. His decision also highlights how much we need more people like him, who give of themselves so that we can learn and, in learning, pay their gift forward. Today, medical schools still need people to donate their bodies so healthy organs can be harvested for the living, so anatomy can be taught to trainee docs, and so the causes and impacts of disease can be better understood.

In first-year medicine, the anatomy department at Dal designated every Friday afternoon as a "living anatomy" session, during which we were introduced to the fine art of physical examination. We were challenged to find the landmarks on the body that could help locate the organs lying beneath. We used each other as models; whichever one of our tablemates drew the short straw would be the model to be poked and prodded the following Friday. It was always a male—women were exempt from being models—and besides, we had only five women in a class of sixty-eight first-year students. When it came to the urogenital exam, the women were plucked from our presence, apparently to be poked and prodded by female professors. At our table, the unfortunate classmate who drew the short straw as model for the male urogenital demonstration had to suffer through a full week of teasing before baring all on Friday. It didn't help our poor classmate when one joker at our table produced a very large magnifying glass just before we started a urogenital exam. The remaining details must remain buried among the ghosts of Dal's anatomy lab.

The deceased can teach us, then, and so can the living. During my undergraduate years at Acadia and then at Dal I befriended Maynard MacAskill, a fellow Cape Bretoner with whom I would remain close for decades. Maynard was preparing to graduate and start practice in the north highlands of the province by the time I arrived at medical school. He introduced me to Arthur Stairs, who had hired Maynard as his caregiver. I would soon recognize Stairs as one of the three wisest men I would meet in my academic life. Stairs (1919–1973) was the scion of a Halifax mercantile and banking family that had been prominent in Halifax since the early 1800s. His ancestor William Stairs founded Wm. Stairs, Son and Morrow, a hardware business, in 1814. Four generations later, in 1935, young Arthur joined the firm he would later lead as president and chairman, but only after serving with distinction in the Royal Canadian Navy during the Second World War. When I met him in 1966, he was still running the business despite suffering from an illness—later diagnosed as Amyotrophic Lateral Sclerosis (ALS), so-called Lou Gehrig's disease—that was gradually paralyzing him.

Maynard suggested I follow him as the live-in caregiver to Arthur but said that I first had to "pass the test"—as he himself had done. He wasn't kidding. Arthur Stairs was no pushover, helpless though he appeared to be on my first visit. I was on edge when I timidly entered his bedroom, which was outfitted with state-of-the-art physiotherapy equipment. Stairs spoke in short, staccato bursts, gasping for air to finish a rasping phrase or a short sentence. Every word was carefully chosen; he had no time or energy to waste on superficial pleasantries. His first question was simple: "What are you reading now?"

Whoa, that took me by surprise. He recognized that immediately. "You can tell a lot by what a man reads," he said. I don't recall what I told him. I was probably reading anatomy textbooks and little else. He guessed as much and said, "You'd better get hold of yourself, and you'd better read more. And you'd better do it while you're with me." As our conversation continued, I began to enjoy our slow-motion give-and-take. And then he told me something I haven't forgotten to this day. "In this job, Stewart, you will be my hands, my feet, and to some degree the rest of my body, but you will NE-VER...BE... MY...BRAIN." Those four words were slow and deliberate, each using up every bit of chest muscle and diaphragm strength left to him to gasp out and emphasize the meaning. I knew, right away, that he was absolutely right.

In that brief encounter, Arthur Stairs taught me one of the most valuable lessons I ever learned during medical school: however disabled the human frame may be, it was the person that mattered, the *whole* person. As Arthur's caregiver during my first year at Dal, I tended to his every bodily need, but in return I received a priceless lesson in humility that was as important as anything I learned in medical school. He repeatedly reminded me that I should understand patients as human beings, not just as "cases." In doing so, he threw cold water on any arrogance I might have felt or developed as a young medical student.

It was my good fortune to meet two other great teachers in those first years of medical school. As rookies, my colleagues and I spent much of our time listening to lectures, which is seldom a blessing. However, Dr. Richard Lorraine de Chasteney Holbourne Saunders,[14] head of the anatomy department, excelled in performing to the dramatic standards implicit in his very name. With his back to the students, red chalk in one hand and blue in the other, he would simultaneously draw the arterial system in red and the venous system in blue. More astoundingly, he delivered a brilliant lecture to the chalkboard and to the room while both hands sketched out the body's architecture. Saunders was the leader of a group of grumpy, eccentric Scots who ruled the roost in the anatomy department. His lectures, in what medical students often considered the most boring of subjects—anatomy—routinely climaxed in standing ovations. A prima donna of the first rank, Saunders would often return to the lecture theatre like a musician bent on performing an encore, bow, and thank us for our generous applause even while his actions prolonged it.

Yes, the man was a ham, but I learned a crucial lesson from him. I was already an experienced public speaker when I entered medical school and had learned a thing or two about engaging an audience. But I was a piker compared to Saunders, and I strove to imitate his skill—and not only at Dal Medicine where I would soon take on leadership positions. Later, in my role as a teacher in medical schools or on hospital wards, I was comfortable in front of students, colleagues, patients, and families. And even later, in electoral politics as in medical politics, I knew I had to engage an audience before trying to secure votes or ask a premier or cabinet for more funding for better healthcare services. Richard Lorraine de Chasteney Holbourne Saunders, for better or worse, helped show me the way.

Early in my Dal years, then, I absorbed important lessons from Stairs the patient and Saunders the performer. But neither would have as much influence on me as Robert (Bob) Scharf,[15] a true trailblazer.

In our first years at Dal, under a forward-looking innovation in the curriculum, medical students were placed in a hospital setting for one week. Some special serendipity was at work when I was assigned to the emergency department at the Victoria General (VG) Hospital, where Scharf practised and taught. Right on time, I entered timidly through the doorway marked "Emergency," clutching my little black bag and outfitted in an overly starched (and scratchy) short white coat, the usual mark of a neophyte medical student. And there he was—the Chief, with his equally starched but *long* white coat wafting behind him, as he half-trotted down the hallway until he spotted…me!

I can remember every detail of my first meeting with him as if it were yesterday. He sprung toward me with a book under one arm and an x-ray under the other. He didn't say, "I'm Bob Scharf." He said, "Come over here. I want to show you something." He picked up the x-ray, put it up on the viewing box and said, "You see that white spot over there? Whatever would you think it is?" I was dumbfounded. I doubt I'd even *seen* an x-ray before; I didn't know whether it was upside down or sideways. But before I could blurt out anything, he answered his own question, in essence adopting his own version of the Socratic method. "You're right! That's exactly what it is—tuberculosis; and don't you ever forget it. It's still around."

Scharf was rare in that he engaged with me as a first-year student instead of just letting me tag along behind him. He took the time to help me figure out what was going on, yet never let me flounder and get flustered. Usually first-year students are ignored, but I had a white coat on and a black bag and that was good enough for him. He asked questions—real questions—but almost always provided us with answers as if we had generated them ourselves. He recognized that a good teacher was a leader, retooling the Socratic questioning in new and imaginative ways, and imprinting on the student's mind not only a fact but a method of reasoning to uncover the fact. Of all the lessons he taught me, that was the one I most used in my medical teaching career. I did my best to pass this insight on to any who came after me.

Bob Scharf took over the emergency department in the first place because he knew the medicine practiced there had to be different, and patients had to be engaged in a different way. He knew, too, that this branch of medicine was like no other, even though, despite its unique nature and requirements, it had yet to be recognized as a specialty. Scharf's re-invention of the emergency department was a master class is healthcare innovation. By the late 1960s, he was sending docs into the sometimes mean streets of Halifax before anyone else had thought of such a notion. As interns serving under his watch, we loved it. We were also working with some very skilled ambulance attendants, thanks to courses Scharf developed for first responders. He sometimes delivered those courses in his own home. We residents quickly recognized how valuable that training was—the ambulance attendants were in many ways better equipped to respond on the scene than we were. We were learning from them, not the other way around.

In the streets we also got to see where patients lived and how they lived. We learned where our patients came from—many were in pretty dire straits when they turned to us for help. These lessons were crucial and unlike any teaching we had received in our early years, both in content and in method. (Bob Scharf will come back into my story later; our lives continued to intertwine, but it must be said it was largely through his lobbying—starting in the 1960s—that the Royal College of Physicians and Surgeons of Canada finally and belatedly recognized Emergency Medicine as a specialty in Canada in the 1980s.)

After my first year of studies, the medical gods favoured me and several of my classmates when we landed coveted jobs at the Victoria General, which included free room and board and ready access to the wards and every nook and cranny in that aging temple of healing. At last! I was to be rescued from the horrors of Howe Hall to something called the Interns' Quarters on University Avenue. "Quarters" was an apt designation. We medical students were often on call and expected to march off to war on the wards—so to speak—at any moment. But we were not being "marched off" to save lives and stamp out disease. Our jobs were far more banal than that. We were on call after 5:00 P.M. to retrieve medical charts of patients who were being seen in the emergency department so that the doctors working there could help sort out what, this time, might be ailing their charges. We would be on call until 7:00 A.M., when the regular medical records staff came on duty. Fortunately, we spent most of our on-call time sleeping, since not all emergency patients had medical histories that had to be reviewed. In reality, the job was pretty cushy and—with perks that included the opportunity to chum around with senior students, residents, and even senior staff members who might come in to see patients prior to their admissions. A major additional benefit was having meals in the dining room of the eight-hundred–bed hospital where, even if the food wasn't quite to one's liking, huge helpings of gossip were available as dessert.

Alas, the job at the hospital was destined to get a tad tougher. The bad news was posted on the Interns' Quarters bulletin board: due to construction of the new pathology building, the aging Interns' Quarters would fall victim to the wrecking ball. And soon. We were shuffled off to live on the twentieth floor of the Park Victoria apartments across the street and up one block from the hospital. Considered at the time to be luxury apartments, the medical school "makeover" to accommodate us managed to transform our digs into a bare and desolate version of a detention centre. There were no blinds on the windows and no furniture except ancient hospital beds with wafer-thin mattresses. In addition, we were compelled to trudge half-conscious to and from the hospital to answer calls of duty in the middle of Halifax winter nights. This was not a trek for the faint of heart. Nor was attempting to sleep with the blinding sun pouring through the windows of the apartment after pulling an all-night shift at the hospital. But we toughed it out through the snowstorms, fog, and damp winter chill of Halifax.

Like soldiers everywhere, our commanding officers—the staff doctors from the hospital—ranged from the mean to the good to the great. Bob Scharf was among the latter. Less gentle men who shall remain unnamed were among the former. The war vets—hardened in the steel of battle—were the toughest of the lot. Some of these senior docs seemed to delight in humiliating and harassing medical students in public—in the cafeteria, in the dining room, on hospital wards. Many members of this untouchable cabal were simply ill-suited to leadership in civilian healthcare. (Since my salad years, this has changed for the better—thanks in large measure to the ascension of women to leadership roles in the field.)

This is not to say I found the traditional hardships of medical schools in that era—the long hours, the poor pay of internship, the need to follow superstar docs on their rounds like so many sheep—to be traumatic. Quite the contrary. Most days, I felt like a kid from "the Mines" who had improbably found his way into medical school and was darned glad to be there. And people stepped up to help me, including Mike MacDonald, a fellow Cape Bretoner and senior administrator at the Victoria General. He was from my hometown of Sydney Mines, and I immediately came to his attention because that's the way it was in those days. If you knew someone, it made a difference. In my second year at Dal, MacDonald hired me for a second job—to stand guard in the medical library after the regular librarian in charge of the journals and medical texts left for the day. It was an ideal time to study, since during the evening very few residents or medical students came near the library. Unfortunately, this easy-sounding job included one odious chore—testing urine samples on every ward of the hospital before the day shifts started. This involved both dipping strips to test urine for sugar levels and other biochemistry, and microscopic tests to check for marauding bacteria. The job stank, literally, and the longer you delayed doing it on any given night, the more it stank. The bouquet of stale urine does not, like that of fine wine, improve with age.

✻

After my second year at Dal, in Canada's Centennial year, 1967, I was to learn another Scharf-like lesson about the value of taking healthcare into communities. I was one among a group of students from across the country who won scholarships to observe the challenges of delivering medical care in the far north of the country, specifically in the Northwest Territories. Our task was to document the levels of hemoglobin in Inuit and other First Nations residents of the Western Arctic, with much of our preparation focussed on study design and logistics.

In retrospect, I feel I should have been embarrassed by my almost total ignorance of life in Canada's north, where Inuit and other Indigenous cultures dated from ancient times. Our briefing meetings in Edmonton prior to the trip attempted to fill in the glaring gaps in our knowledge of the people and their lives. At the beginning of the seminar, we were housed in a large residential facility that also served as a school for Indigenous youth from kindergarten to high school. During the month of August, it was almost completely empty save for our eighty-four–member delegation of medical students from across Canada. We were told all Indigenous students from the residential school were sent back to their families "on the land" during summer break. They would be returning just before the first snows in September. Some of our discussions centred around the idea of separating children—particularly very young children—from their parents for months at a time and then returning them to nomadic life on the land in the short Artic summer. It was not until decades later that I began to recognize the serious implications of putting the lives of Indigenous children into the hands of clergymen who—to put it mildly—did not always honour the trust placed in them. (More than fifty years later, as I write this, Canada is still coming to grips with the tragic story of how badly Indigenous children were abused in residential schools.)

After flying to Inuvik, the largest community in the Northwest Territories, we fanned out to smaller villages and camps throughout the Western Arctic. There we were billeted in remote nursing stations to carry out our research project. Travel was frequently by air and then by canoe or motorboat to small groups of Inuit. Although I had been baptized already by the hordes of blackflies on the Saint John and Mira Rivers, nothing prepared me for the unspeakable attacks of northern blackflies in the Arctic bush. I begin to itch all over and break out in a cold sweat just thinking about the tiny pests. Still, everyone in our group adapted to the routines of the nursing stations, where we enjoyed great hospitality and benefitted from the example of medical people totally dedicated to the people they served.

Back at Dalhousie, I was bitten by the political bug again and ran for the presidency of the Dalhousie Medical Students' Society for the 1968–69 academic year. After a successful campaign, I took off running with the help of a strong executive and the president of our "Class of 1970," Dan Reid. In 1969, we launched what turned into an annual fundraiser, an auction for Foster Parents Plan of Canada (now Plan Canada). Most of our auctioned items were donated by local businesses and medical school departments. The most sought-after item—fetching $400—was an "authentic" lateral x-ray film of Marilyn Monroe's chest. (*O tempora! O mores!*) The donor (a radiology resident) swore it was a copy of the original he obtained while on rotation at a Boston hospital. Our plastic surgeons donated ten lessons in suturing, the hospital cooks their finest version of a birthday cake for ten students, and the dean donated a dinner at a fine Halifax restaurant. The income from the auction enabled us to sponsor not one but ten international foster children.

Flushed with the success of our Foster Parents Plan fundraiser, we decided to live up to the "charity begins at home" maxim by raising funds for local social action groups. The strategy here was to tap into the musical and artistic talents of our medical students. Born of this assumption was *Euphoria!*, a popular annual variety show (which, incidentally, is still running). The show, which often included risqué material that was sometimes tut-tutted by medical school deans, proved too popular to restrain. Tickets to the event at Dalhousie's Rebecca Cohn Auditorium sold out every year it was staged live. Over the years, the event has raised millions of dollars for charities. In 2019, I re-engaged with *Euphoria!* for its golden (fiftieth) anniversary. We set a goal of raising $50,000 for the event—"Fifty for Fifty" was the slogan, and I wrung contributions out of every university campus in Nova Scotia as well as every MD class from the past fifty years and numerous healthcare organizations. They all chipped in, and we readily reached the "Fifty for Fifty" mark within a week.

Of course, 1969 was a remarkable year, not only for the Dalhousie Medical School but for humankind. On July 20, 1969, millions of people gathered around their televisions to watch two American astronauts do something no one had done before. Wearing bulky space suits, Neil Armstrong and Edwin "Buzz" Aldrin became the first human beings to walk on the moon. At that moment, I was treating an elderly patient in a glassed-in atrium while the light from the moon shone down upon us. A black-and-white TV was broadcasting the story. When Neil Armstrong uttered those famous words, "That's one small step for man, one giant leap for mankind," my index finger was inserted into the rectum of my poor patient, probing for the tumor that would soon kill him. The digital examination was by the book, but totally unnecessary. I should have known, and some part of me did know, that my patient's disease was terminal. His death two days later taught me another lesson in humility. Sometimes, it is kinder to not treat patients but rather to let life and death take their course. To many outsiders, practising medicine often seems as dramatic and exciting as walking on the moon. At rare moments, it is just that. Most of the time, it is about being human and striving to do the job while being kind in the process. The patient died two days later. When I met with the family, I told them their loved one and I had watched the moon landing together.

During my term as president of the Medical Students' Society, the other grand event of the academic year was the opening of the Student Union Building (SUB) in November 1968. The SUB celebration launch, held over a three-day period starting November 6, featured student and other exhibits. Our medical society's exhibit focussed on the "new and exciting" developments in healthcare. We decided that, given the prominence of sexually transmitted infections in the port city of Halifax, we should have a special section of our display highlighting contraception and safe sex. We expected this might rock the establishment a bit. Yes, Pierre Trudeau had famously said in 1967, when he served as federal justice minister, that there is "no place for the state in the bedrooms of the nation." But it wasn't until 1969, the year after Trudeau became prime minister, that birth control was legalized in Canada as part of an omnibus justice bill that also authorized therapeutic abortions and decriminalized homosexual acts between consenting adults. Suffice to say that our little information booth at the SUB was not only controversial but arguably illegal—a fact not lost on my fellow student Vonda Hayes. Looking back at the event, Vonda told me she was definitely "voluntold" to staff the booth and was concerned about the perils of a possible police raid, a likely cease-and-desist order from the courts, or at least a slap on the wrist by university administrators. Happily, she was not censured. Mind you, Dr. Vonda did endure years of good-natured teasing as the reputed "contraceptive lady." She never tired of reminding me that I had put her in harm's way. Nor did she regret running the booth. Decades later, she also reminded me that her work there was a public service of the highest order. The purpose, after all, was counselling students about healthy sexual practices.

My presidential responsibilities faded quickly as we began the gradual transition from bookish wide-eyed students to the sudden shock of the reality of bedside medicine, surgical clinics, and operating rooms. For me, that transition had a soft landing. Being a caregiver to Art

Stairs had prepared me for much of what I later faced in clinics or on the wards. I came out of that experience appreciating the fundamentals of patient care beyond the skilled suturing of a wound or even identification of the subtle signs of tuberculosis on an x-ray. But I needed a broader experience within a clinical setting before I would be let loose on the wards. That opportunity came in 1968, toward the end of my third academic year, when I learned about the potential for medical students to apply for positions as orderlies on the clinical wards at the Victoria General. Orderlies were the equivalent of caregivers working under the direct supervision of senior nurses, and with my record of work with Art Stairs, I was well-positioned to get the position—which I did. So, at the beginning of that summer I set off from the Interns' Quarters in overly starched white pants and smock to take up duties as assigned on the neurosurgical ward, located in what was called "the Pavilion." That part of the hospital was a holdover from its construction in 1922 as the "Private Pavilion"—for paying patients only in those pre-medicare days.

Working in the neurosurgical unit prodded me into a review of neuroanatomy. I never thought I'd go back to such torture, but I must admit it was a boon. I got into a routine of choosing a patient's chart, reading the residents' and nurses' notes, and then researching the anatomy and care related to the patient's needs. The clinical bedside care I was expected to provide was an easy transition from my time with Arthur Stairs. He had indeed taught me well. The summer on that ward was a major boost for my morale as well; I began to feel that the decision I had made years ago in the cloistered cushion of Acadia was the right one. I could scarcely wait to get on with it.

I didn't have to wait long. The Christmas holidays were fast-approaching in 1969, and I was looking forward to getting back to the island for some snowshoeing in the Highlands, or being stuffed with Mom's caloric goodies—preferably both. That was, until I was approached by one of Dal's rising stars, Dr. Reg Yabsley, at the time a newly arrived Dalhousie graduate in orthopaedic surgery who had completed post-graduate training in Toronto and Europe. He had risen rapidly in the ranks and begun as head of the new Division of Orthopaedic Surgery. I had only occasionally met him during my time on the neurosurgery wards and immediately took a liking to him. He was warm, personable, generous with his time for students, and always respectful of nurses and OR staff (often a revealing test of any physician). Possibly because of my ubiquitous presence in the hospital and neurosurgical ward that summer, he suggested I might visit him in his office and discuss possibly helping him over the upcoming Christmas holidays. During that time, the ranks of house staff (specialty residents-in-training) were thinned out. To accommodate the sudden decrease in staff, patients who could be discharged were, and staff physicians took up the slack. Occasionally, senior medical students were offered "junior resident" positions, with obligations tailored to their level of training. We were qualified to perform routine work on the wards or assist during surgeries. These positions were few, and limited to fourth-year students. His offer to me was unexpected, but I quickly put aside any thoughts of the winter wonders of the Highlands and signed up with Dr. Yabsley. My experience with him stood out as my first *real* introduction to what my future in medicine could be. I could scarcely have even wished for a gentler entry to the world of medical practice and for a better guide. As a teacher, he was skilled and effective; as a physician he was a top-notch clinician and deft surgeon; as a *human* he was outstandingly compassionate, long-suffering, and kind. He set a standard to aspire to, if not reach.

The final year of our MD education was designed to prepare us for general practice or to choose a specialty. Internship was all about delivering hands-on patient care while being held accountable to senior staff. I had the opportunity to do a rotation in obstetrics at a regional hospital located in the town of Truro, about a hundred kilometres (sixty miles) north of Halifax. This would be the closest I would come to independent practice since I was the only intern on duty twenty-four hours a day—reporting to GPs or obstetricians. In reality, I found myself learning most of the hands-on obstetrical care routines from the nurses. I soon recognized they knew their stuff, many through the grit of experience, and many because they had been through the test of childbirth themselves. They were also willing to share their practical experience and wisdom of the years with me. This experience was a welcome contrast to my experience on the wards of the Halifax teaching hospitals, where medical students were often considered nuisances from whom patients had to be sheltered. I also learned early on in my experience in Truro that childbirth was mainly an exercise in waiting and worrying, while the patients did the work. The medical team's focus was simple and our goals—a satisfied mom and a healthy baby—were clear.

I spent so much time waiting with mothers-to-be that I decided to learn to play ukulele. I drew on my past musical interests, learned a few chords, and was soon ready for my premiere performance. The "singing intern" seemed to be a popular addition to life on the obstetrical ward of the Colchester County Hospital. This brief flirtation with minor fame aside, I learned that music can uplift the spirits of healthcare staff and patients. I suspected then what research would later show—live performances (and live performing) have a therapeutic effect. The integration of music—and arts generally—and medical school curricula would become an abiding passion for me in later years.

My connection with the hospital in Truro wasn't entirely severed when I left for Halifax. I had the met an engaging and attractive nurse during an attempted resuscitation of a patient in the cardiac care unit. We connected immediately, and the news that she was preparing to take a job at the Victoria General set my imagination soaring. The woman (whose privacy I will protect) and I were attracted to each other; we shared interests and initially felt we wanted to spend our lives together. Alas, the relationship was not destined to endure, as my story will show.

In my fifth and final year at Dalhousie, as I took part in Dalhousie's rotating internship program, I would learn a hard and memorable lesson in psychiatry. A few patients in the service became so attached to me that they sought me out after I had left. At least one tracked me to distant Neils Harbour in northern Cape Breton after I had set up in family medicine in a remote part of the island. I hadn't thought I was devoting too much attention to patients on the psychiatry ward, but something wasn't quite kosher. I sought out the advice of a psychiatrist whose opinion I would respect and advice I would readily accept. The lesson learned? Patients are your patients, not your friends and that line must neither be crossed nor be seen to be crossed.

My decision to set up my medical shop back home on the island in Neils Harbour drove me to prepare for the eventual move with a feverish intensity. In my last year at medical school, I was obsessed with hitting the ground running in my first foray into medicine as a general practitioner, and that meant absorbing knowledge and—more importantly—learning through experience. I put in every extra minute of time I could with Bob Scharf in the emergency department, caring for patients and watching and learning as other doctors plied their trade. I was also spending less and less time with the nurse I had met a month earlier but who prophetically enough showed no inclination to travel to a remote part of Cape Breton Island with me. This, despite the fact that going to Neils Harbour was much like going home for me. By practising there, I would be honouring a commitment to Maynard MacAskill—who finished a few years ahead of me in medical school and had gone to Neils Harbour (on the island we both called home)— to serve as a community doc.

During the months I spent preparing for my future with Bob Scharf in the emergency department, we came to an understanding that I would spend at least two years in the north Highlands and then consider getting a residency in emergency medicine—wherever he could find an academically credible program. We more or less formalized this plan with a handshake, and I considered the deal done. The "when" of the deal was the major unknown. I was unaware that he had already begun petitioning the Royal College that they begin immediately to define a specialty called "Emergency Medicine" and that he would be happy to volunteer to do some preparatory work for their deliberations. He was one of the first in Canada to formally propose this, but before any progress was made, I was packing my bags and heading off to the island—and whatever awaited me in the land of the eagle and the moose.

CHAPTER 4

INTO THE WILDERNESS, 1970-1972

WHAT AWAITED ME IN THE LAND OF THE EAGLE AND THE MOOSE, AS IT TURNED OUT, WERE a seagull and a cat. The cat in question had a fishhook stuck in its tongue. The seagull was suffering from a broken wing. Both creatures were among my first patients at the Highlands Medical Clinic in Neils Harbour, Cape Breton, where the doctor also served as veterinarian, dentist, pharmacist, ambulance driver, occasional gravedigger, and coroner. A couple of local lads brought the huge black cat, fishhook and all, into the hospital—and it was no salmon angler's delicate hook. It was a cod hook, big enough to catch and hold a species that can easily weigh eighty pounds at maturity. The cat, draped over one of the boy's arms, was so still I thought it was dead. But no, the cat was breathing, if almost dead from starvation. Euthanasia was perhaps one option. But one look at the boys' sad but hopeful faces and I knew I'd make a bad start in my new practice by killing the cat.

Of course, I had neither training nor experience as a vet. Happily, Nelda McLeod—a veteran nurse who had served in the clinic for decades, took charge. "Don't worry, Doctor dear, we can do this all right," she told me. "Now, you go get some gauze and a garbage bag and I'll go get the ether can."

"Ether?" I asked.

"That's right. We don't use it all that much anymore, but we keep it around, you know."

Nelda then offered a step-by-step guide to removing a cod hook from a cat's tongue. The boys were to put the cat on a stretcher. Nelda was to thoroughly soak the gauze pads in ether and toss them into the garbage bag. I was to wrestle the big black cat into the garbage bag. And so it went. Sure enough, the cat settled down after causing a bit of a commotion. Nelda then thrust a pair of pliers into my hands and told me to get on with the job. "Doctor, you've got about three minutes." I extracted the cod hook with more speed than skill, then looked on in horror as the re-awakened cat—freed from the bag—shot off like a thunderbolt, jumping on patients' beds and generally running amok until we could corner the frenzied feline. We kept the three of them— two boys and one revived cat—for the afternoon and made sure the trio was well fed. So my first patient was a "cure" and the importance of teamwork in medicine was amply demonstrated! (The seagull story was just as dramatic. Suffice it to say it was treated and returned to the wild—or at least to the nearby fishing wharf where it could forage for scraps from the local fleet.)

Why the work as a vet? Well, in that spring of 1970, the Neils Harbour hospital served a remote rural area in Scottish-style highlands, and there were too few healthcare services in the area. We delivered healthcare to most of Victoria County's eight thousand or so souls, spread out over 2,500 square kilometres (1,000 square miles) of territory traversed by narrow, treacherous mountain roads. The nearest full-service hospitals were located in Sydney, a hundred-mile drive away. We docs served as jacks of all medical trades. I had made a couple of trial runs home to the island to work with Maynard MacAskill before setting up shop as a fully-fledged doc, but nothing had really prepared me for remote rural practice. (To further complicate matters, Dr. MacAskill welcomed my arrival as an opportunity to depart for off-island vacations. Maynard needed an extended break, and he took it.)

The area's economy depended on the three *F*s—fishing, forestry, and farming—with a *T* thrown in for tourism during the brief but glorious summers. Adult literacy rates were low; experience and common sense were seen as more valuable than book learning or educational levels. In the early 1970s, physicians—and members of clergy—were seen and treated as a breed apart. Not quite deities, but not "one of us" either. Certainly, you didn't ask the doc or a minister of the cloth to share a beer with you. I was too busy in the practice to feel lonely, but I sure knew I was isolated. Working alone at the clinic—or travelling for hours to house calls—represented a dramatic departure from the collaborative (and often supervised) medical care I had provided to patients at the big teaching hospital in Halifax.

Luckily, Public Health nurse Isabel MacDonald often rushed to my rescue in this brave new world. Her knowledge of North Highlands history, families, and culture was encyclopedic. If the Jones family in Ingonish had a history of heart disease, she could track it back three generations. If the patriarch of the MacDonald clan up on North Mountain turned mean after a few snorts of rum, she'd sound a warning for me. She knew where the roads were dangerous and the ice was thin (so to speak). Most importantly, she taught me that a doctor's house call was also a social event. I should expect to be offered a cup of tea and a biscuit with butter after the clinical part of the visit was done, and I should darned well sit down to my tea.

I was also fortunate to strike close friendships with David Reid, an Acadia classmate, and his wife, Patti. David, the priest at Saint Andrew's Anglican Church in Neils Harbour, was a willing assistant in my medical adventures. If a patient was suffering his last illness as home, my job was to treat him while he was breathing, pronounce him dead as county coroner if he stopped, and remove the body as a primitive version of an ambulance attendant. David often accompanied me on house calls to provide pastoral care, and also to help me haul the dead out of their homes. After one brutal blizzard, we briefly lost a poor departed soul (wrapped in a makeshift white shroud) in a deep pile of fluffy snow. David and I had to dig him out of that hole, and later bury him in another. The gravedigger's job was formally assigned to our elderly caretaker at Buchanan Memorial Hospital, a fourteen-bed facility located next to our medical clinic. But the gentleman in question suffered from arthritis, and it was often left to David and me to do his job. Neils Harbour is built largely on solid rock (Devonian granite), so the job was difficult in summer and all but impossible in winter after the ground froze. The all-season solution was to deploy a pneumatic drill to excavate graves for the dearly departed. (Dynamite might have come in handy, but we had no ready supply.) I would tease my friend, the Reverend David, by accusing him of keeping the drill just inside the main entry of the church simply to remind us all of our mortality!

Given David's role in my practice, I could hardly refuse his request to play the organ at his Christmas eve service in 1970, and therein lies of tale of several malfunctioning organs. The church's long-serving but long-defunct pipe organ was a victim of the frigid winter in the usually unheated church building by the ocean. It was essentially unusable, even for a fake organist like me. But some years before my arrival on the musical scene of Neils Harbour, an ancient and ailing pump organ had been pressed into service. That ancient instrument was in bad shape, having developed a bad case of the blind staggers accompanied by serious wheezing. Its bellows were leaky and Hercules himself couldn't keep enough air in them to make a decent sound. So as a matter of self-preservation, I suggested to David in November that we travel to Sydney and rent a small Hammond organ for the upcoming Christmas Eve service, which we did. I practised and even mostly mastered the one-octave bass pedals. By mid-December I was ready and eager. What I hadn't figured into the musical equation was the harsh and unforgiving North Highlands winter.

Christmas Eve arrived. The picturesque Anglican church overlooking the snow-covered rocky coastline was resplendent in the glow of

Christmas candles. Everything was ready—or so it seemed. But early in the afternoon of December 24, one of the worst blizzards of the season buried us in heavy, clinging snow. We could usually handle snow; the single power line over Cape Smokey couldn't. That's what caused us grief. Even before the first strains of "Silent Night" sounded, off went the power and our beloved borrowed electric organ fell silent.

My solution seemed simple enough: I recruited a young lad to pump the pedals on the old church organ. I had seen this kid around the village, but he was never a patient of mine. No matter, his job was to hide under the organ bench and push the pedals for all his worth with his arms, while I attempted a repertoire of Christmas carols. Sadly, my volunteer organ-pumper seemed to be as inept at pumping as I was as an organist. He was failing so much at the job as the service progressed that I finally bent down to see what could be wrong, only to discover that his lips were a ghastly shade of blue and he was clearly short of breath. I immediately recognized the third organ failure of the night, and this one was deadly serious. The lad, who always seemed "a bit off" to use the parlance of the day, likely had an undiagnosed heart problem. I loaded him into my Jeep and headed off into the night toward our wee hospital just outside the village. He quickly recovered once his organ-pumping duties were halted, but as soon as the roads were cleared over the mountain on Boxing Day, we headed in my trusty Jeep to the children's hospital in Halifax, some five hundred kilometres (three hundred miles) south. I delivered him into the care of the cardiac team at one of the teaching hospitals I had left just months earlier. Then I crossed the street to the Interns' Quarters and slept like a baby as the surgeons corrected the boy's heart defect. (Fifty years later, this same fellow—grown into a giant of a man—approached me in the Co-op store during one of my frequent visits to the North Highlands to offer his thanks. I'm not sure I fully deserved it, given the risk I exposed him to under the organ bench.)

To say the least, our medical practice was a diverse one. The one task I was quite unprepared for was dealing with the epidemic of dental decay, in which tooth extraction was assigned to docs in rural areas devoid of real dentists. At the time, extraction was included on the so-called fee schedule for Nova Scotia doctors, which meant the government paid for the service under the province's medicare program. The affluent or the wise might have preferred paying a real dentist in nearby Baddeck to do the work; the rest were all too happy to seek out my services. My colleague Maynard had forewarned me about this work, and I prepared in two ways: Before heading north to the practice, I sat in on the early Dalhousie dental school lectures to learn the rudimentary rules of extraction and administering nerve blocks, and I purchased a real dentist chair and other equipment from the widow of a deceased practitioner.

Turns out I applied my dentistry skills with a little too much enthusiasm—largely because I didn't want to cause undue pain to anyone—and figured if a little lidocaine was good, a lot of lidocaine was better. The bad news was that I administered so much of it in the early days that patients would experience prolonged loss of sensation and nerve function and would end up walking around with numb or crooked smiles for hours or even days. The worse news was that patients loved this approach. One local gossip spread the word, with a marked physician-induced lisp: "That Dr. Stewart sure knows what he's doing. He doesn't spare the freezing and I didn't feel a thing for a whole week!" This mantra made my dental services all the more popular—though I soon adapted my practice to the realization that a little lidocaine goes a long way.

My dad also played a role in the delivery of dental services. Always eager and able to help, he decided to plumb the dentist chair to get what was called the "swishy thing" (the rinse basin) to work. It would be the crowning achievement of my dental practice. Easy work for a man as handy with a welding torch as Dad, but unfortunately the venue was not a coal mine but a prefab building shipped by boat to the northland and insulated with straw. As he deployed his welding torch under the floor of the building, which sat above the ground, he protected the straw from fire by placing a couple of large cardboard boxes between the torch and the highly flammable insulation. This worked like a charm until Dad threw the boxes into the alleyway after the job was done. The minute they hit the open air, oxygen did its work and the cardboard burst into flame. Yes, we did have a local fire truck. No, it was not useful. In those days, it was parked in Tommy Turner's yard and had no wheels. Fortunately, we successfully fought the fire with a garden hose, so there was no property damage, but my hopes for dental fame went up in smoke.

My early experiences in veterinary medicine and dentistry feel more like farce than tragedy in the retelling, but in truth the job involved dealing with a great deal of heartbreak and death, and the consequences of grinding poverty. In the first months of my practice, I was seeing a patient (I'll call her Maggie) in the clinic who had travelled from Bay St. Lawrence, a thirty-mile drive away over perilous mountain roads, to see me about her blood pressure problem. She had a large family, and it was hard for her to get away. Unfortunately, I heard my ring—the doctor's ring—on our party line in Neils Harbour and I had to take the call. (There were five rings on the party line—one for the hospital, one for the lab/x-ray technician, one for the clinic, one for the doctor's house, and one for the Anglican priest.) The caller was an RCMP constable who said a pickup truck had gone off a cliff on a mountain road past Meat Cove. Death would have to be pronounced at the scene on Bear Mountain before the body of the victim could be moved. He said the coroner would have to travel to the accident scene. Of course, I was the coroner, as my caller knew all too well.

I abandoned poor Maggie and jumped into my Jeep station wagon, which served as a makeshift ambulance. (My dad had drilled holes in

the floor of the vehicle to secure a hospital stretcher in place with bolts.)
At the scene, I could see the truck was hung up on an outcrop over
the cliff. It turned out there had been three people in the truck, two
men and a woman. They'd been drinking after returning from one of
the stills that peppered the mountainside above. The men were able to
scramble up the cliff and summon help. The RCMP were pretty certain
the woman was dead but couldn't move her from the truck until the
coroner saw her. The crew had rigged up a system of ropes they tied
around my torso to lower me into the truck. "Don't worry, we'll do our
best to hang on tight," said one constable, smiling wryly. (In tough circumstances, medical humour is often healing, or at least relieving.) The
woman was indeed dead. Eventually, we were both hauled up the cliff
and I was able to take the body away, as a proper coroner, in my Jeep.

Unfortunately, the circumstances surrounding Maggie's follow-up
visit were even more tragic. Again, I was talking to her in my office in a
continuing battle to control her severe hypertension. Again, there came
the doctor's office ring from the hospital. It was the RCMP again—a
double drowning to deal with. Two brothers, aged fifteen and sixteen,
had lost their lives in a lake near Bay St. Lawrence. The constable on
the phone told me the names of both the parents; the father was with
them; his wife, Maggie, was with me! I told Maggie she'd have to stay
until I came back from the accident because her blood pressure was
way too high, but I didn't tell her the details I knew. Before I headed
to Bay St. Lawrence I took Maggie over to the hospital, where I told
the nurse to isolate her in the small delivery room until I returned
and not allow anyone to see her except staff. Eventually I returned to
Neils Harbour with the bodies of the two boys laid out in the back of
my Jeep. When I told Maggie about the deaths of her sons, she barely
batted an eyelash. This was what I expected, given the stoic character
of the people in the North Highlands. When she eventually did shed
a few tears, the nurses in attendance broke down completely in that
tiny little room. I left to take yet another phone call, or I would have
joined them in expressing the grief we all felt.

We had four drowning deaths in the North Highlands in that summer of 1970, and I realized that very few people in our area could swim, despite the extensive coastline and dozens of beautiful inland lakes and rivers. Local lore suggested that fishermen didn't learn to swim because they thought it was bad luck if you swam away from your boat. They would be unlikely to take lessons. For kids, swimming wasn't part of the culture. They would go fishing in the middle of a river, standing in waders in running water up to their waists, but they wouldn't dream of taking a swimming lesson. I wasn't about to give up on the kids, though. I threatened them, saying if they didn't take the lessons from the Red Cross that their next immunization shot would be administered through the biggest needle they ever saw. I coerced them and threatened them, which was quite unprofessional, but I was facing a situation that I didn't recall anyone speaking about in our discussions of medical ethics at Dalhousie.

Nor did medical school prepare me for what happened on the highway near "Little Smokey" on the night of April 26, 1971, about a year after I first moved to Neils Harbour.

A dramatic costal promontory known simply in Cape Breton as Cape Smokey marks the entrance to the area where I lived and practised. South of Smokey you could find "civilization"; north of it you were in wilderness. Drivers heading north on Route 30 have to navigate their vehicles up the mountain toward Cape Smokey via a switchback highway featuring grades so steep that travellers feel as if they are ascending directly into the heavens. In winter, the mountain can easily become a barrier. If the weather is bad or the roads have iced up, only a brave or foolish driver will risk driving north toward the resort town of Ingonish. Beyond Ingonish, the highway climbs "Little Smokey" toward our clinic and hospital at Neils Harbour. Once you've climbed

Smokey itself, you've entered the country that local people call "down North"—a universe unto itself.

It was in this territory, south of Neils Harbour, that I was summoned late in the evening to a house call in Ingonish at the request of a seventy-something woman. She said she was calling on behalf of her mother, who was a few years shy of one hundred years old. I had a visitor staying with me, Ken Murray, a close friend from medical school and now in his final years of training. "Mummy" had fallen from a plum tree the previous fall, fracturing her hip. Her daughter, the truly apprehensive member of the small household, made frequent calls to the clinic, begging a doctor to come see her mother at all hours of the day and night. Answering the call on that fateful April day was a wearying but necessary part of my duty of care, and off I went. The visit was uneventful and was more of a social call, even at that hour of the night. The patient was consulted; comforting words were spoken; tea was served, and I headed toward home into the teeth of a not-unusual spring blizzard as darkness approached.

In Ingonish, I checked in as I often did at the detachment of the Royal Canadian Mounted Police (RCMP). I sometimes slept there on the way back from house calls to avoid treacherous weather or driving while fatigued in the dark. The officers on duty gave me clear advice—the storm is worsening, don't drive home tonight. Despite that, I decided to return to Neils Harbour. Maynard was off duty the next day, and I needed to be there to do rounds on the patients with him and Ken in tow. At Little Smokey, with my windshield wipers losing the battle to clear the snow in the darkness, I veered off the right side of the road toward a cliff that descended toward the Atlantic Ocean. RCMP later said a moose on the road—a common sight in that part of the island—may have prompted me to swerve. That can never be known for certain, although rumour had it that suspicious bits of moose hair were found embedded in the wreck of my beloved Jeep. I do know, though, that I wouldn't have lived to tell this story had I left the highway in a more dangerous area, where the cliffs drop more steeply to the ocean.

Duty staff at the hospital in Neils Harbour were anxiously awaiting my return, and were quick to call the RCMP station in Ingonish when I didn't turn up. The Mounties immediately set out into the storm on snowmobiles, only to reluctantly turn around when the search was deemed too dangerous to conduct in the worsening weather. Later, they told me the turnaround point was only a hundred or so metres from the scene of the accident. Luckily, I was saved by two guardian angels. The first was Ken Murray, who would later follow me into practice at Neils Harbour and stay there for half a century. Ken had urged me to wear a big winter parka on the drive to and from my house call. He had also decided, wisely enough, to stay in Neils Harbour rather than join me on the journey. If I hadn't been wearing that jacket when the accident occurred, the hypothermia with which I was inevitably afflicted would likely have killed me.

My second angel was a fisherman travelling the next morning to a nearby wharf to see if his vessel was safe in the wake of the storm. He spotted the place where my Jeep had left the road and alerted the RCMP. I blush to confess I don't recall the fisherman's name (if I ever knew it) and have been unable to track him down. Indeed, what happened that day and in the months of rehabilitation that followed are largely lost to my memory. I suffered a brain injury during the crash, and I am only able to tell the story through the recollections of others—and by reviewing my medical charts.

Here's what happened next, according to my charts and third-party accounts. An ambulance was summoned—it was newly acquired and the result of a vigorous effort by many of us to set up the service. I was taken to Neils Harbour, where it was quickly decided to pack me off to Sydney City Hospital. Frank Kelly was the senior surgeon there. A frontal-temporal lobe injury was suspected even as it quickly worsened. In the warmth of the hospital setting, the body rewarms, and injured brain tissue begins to swell, so the fear was I likely had an expanding bleed. The treatment for this was clear—bore a hole in the skull to relieve the pressure. Kelly made the appropriate diagnosis under the circumstances—and there was no time to lose. "I can't do this here," he told his team. "We have to call neurosurgery [in Halifax]."

The decision was made to send me by ambulance toward Halifax, where a young and adventurous neurosurgeon named Rollie Langille had been consulted. I use the word "toward" advisedly, for Rollie had hatched a plan to jump into his car and drive to the hospital in Antigonish, where he could treat me sooner; all he would need was a sterile brace and a bit. Antigonish is located about halfway between Sydney and Halifax, and he wanted to meet me there, at St. Martha's Hospital. When we arrived in Antigonish, Rollie hadn't yet arrived at the hospital, and my attendants decided to speed on toward Halifax rather than wait around. Rollie, not known for his slow and careful driving, was indeed zipping down the road toward Antigonish. The ambulance attendants, not recognizing his car, sped to Halifax at well over any legal speed limits, but Rollie wasn't to be outdone. He passed the ambulance, did a quick U-turn, and floored his long-suffering car, arriving at the Victoria General about five minutes after the ambulance.

At the Victoria General Hospital, where I had spent so much time as a student, the medical team knew it was touch and go—a brain injury poses a genuine threat to life. The diagnostic tools available to the neurosurgeons in the early 1970s were nothing like we have today—there were no CT scans, no computers or digital imaging which now enable us to do so much more. The diagnostic tool at the time was a primitive one by today's standards, but still could be useful. A special radioactive dye injected into the vein could collect in areas of the brain that were bleeding. Most of the time, blood clotting outside the brain's vessels could be distinguished from a diffuse radioactivity within brain tissue. The doctors who read the scan saw that the area of radioactivity was diffuse, not concentrated. They concluded, rightly, that a clot hadn't formed and there was a good chance I would survive the accident. Given that diagnosis, there was no need to drill burr holes into my skull and relieve pressure or tie off bleeding vessels. I remember none of this, but I was able to put together the story from reading the nursing observations and physicians' progress notes, which said I was largely unresponsive at the time. The medical chart also showed hypertonic saline and mannitol (a sugar molecule) were administered to lower pressure on the brain and draw fluid out of brain tissue.

I was not a happy camper or a model patient when I was moved to the neuro ward and then to the Nova Scotia Rehabilitation Centre. I had right-sided paralysis with very limited function in my right leg and not much more in my arm. The physiotherapists were charged with helping me maintain muscle tone and bulk and then restore function. I resisted their assistance—and detested their persistence. I would cling to the bed rails with my "good" arm when they came to fetch me and throw childlike tantrums to try to avoid the therapy. (My injured frontal lobe wasn't very good at controlling my resentment at being made to do things I didn't want to—and couldn't—do.) They were asking me to accomplish the impossible as far as I was concerned. As I gradually improved, I also learned how difficult and frustrating it can be as a patient on the other side of the blanket from a team of physicians with interns and residents trailing them sheepishly, as I had done. I had to use a wheelchair for some weeks, and my impression was that none of the dozens of physicians who talked to me during that period ever attempted to make eye contact. All of the white coats would stand around me while I was sitting in a wheelchair and unable to raise my face upward with my neck collar on. I ended up answering or asking questions while talking at their crotches! The situation so infuriated me that I later wrote an editorial—or should I say a lamentation—entitled "Conversations with Crotches." (It was too angry by half, and I am happy I resisted the temptation to send it off for publication in the *Journal of the Canadian Medical Association*.)

During rehab, I had a bigger concern than right-side paralysis. What worried me most was the loss of my ability to speak. I was experiencing what's called "expressive aphasia" or Broca's aphasia, which meant I knew what I wanted to say but couldn't say it. Every other day, I would be taken to the Izaak Walton Killam Hospital for Children to meet with the therapists, an excursion that gave me a chance to sit on the floor and play with some of the kids. That I enjoyed, though I'm sure not all the parents were happy with the situation. The therapists taught me some coping skills that would prove useful for the rest of my life. Slowing down my speech was one. Holding my hand in front of my face to mask lingering self-consciousness about my facial movements was another. One speech therapist prescribed *Peanuts* comics to address a real cognitive challenge—I couldn't follow a storyline very well. She started by asking me to read three-panel comics, the kind published every day in the newspapers. Then I moved up to six- or eight-panel comics from the pen of the legendary Charles M. Schulz. Next, it was book-length stories featuring Linus, Snoopy, Charlie, and the whole bunch. It's no exaggeration to say Charlie Brown helped restore me—body, brain, and soul.

My rehabilitation period was one of the oddest times of my life. I existed in a sort of liminal twilight zone. To this day, I can't define the boundary between what I recall and what people told me about that period. I was also labile—inwardly furious with physicians and physios one minute, playing with kids and reading the funnies the next. My brain injury also left me feeling apathetic about what were formerly some of my most significant relationships. I was nonchalant, vaguely whimsical about my life and prospects. I was told my fiancée, for instance, visited me less and less frequently as my rehab period progressed. Ho-hum, I thought. By July of that year, the relationship had essentially died, and I was gut-aching to get out of Halifax and back to Neils Harbour. I probably left the rehab centre before I was ready to re-enter the world, but I was determined to deliver medical care as a doc rather than endure it any longer as a patient, so back to Cape Breton I went.

I did take a lingering deficit back with me to the North Highlands Medical Clinic. It wasn't about my right-side paralysis, which was treated successfully by those courageous physiotherapists whose help I so vigorously spurned. I still felt some weakness on my right side, particularly when I was tired, but it wasn't visible to others and since I was only thirty-one years of age I was quickly regaining strength. Nor did I suffer from any cognitive difficulties—my mind was as sharp as ever—or as dull, if you prefer. What persisted were problems communicating; I spoke hesitantly and sometimes stuttered.

At the same time, the patient load was shifting back toward Maynard, a reversal of my early months in the area, when some patients tend to "try out" the new doc and compare notes. Maynard was also used to solo practice, keeping strict hours in the clinic; he kept his patient visits short and to the point. He was an expert organizer—a trait in solo practice that is beneficial to everyone, doc and patient alike. That didn't make him any less effective or any less skilled as a practitioner or diagnostician—he was a great country doc, and I learned a great deal from him. I give credit to Maynard in large measure for my ability later in my residency years in Los Angeles and then in my leadership roles in medicine.

My approach, as a new physician to the area, was more methodical than his. For better or worse, I spent more time with patients, extended my clinic hours to meet their needs, and was seen by some as more sympathetic. But that approach drained me, and slowly tried my patience and diminished my empathy. After my return to the clinic, one of the nurses confirmed what I suspected. Patients were avoiding me. They'd call and ask which doctor was "on" and were more likely to show up when Maynard was working. Just like the poor kid I'd trapped under the organ bench on Christmas Eve, I was seen as "a little off." It was unfair to Maynard and to the practice to continue, and I decided it was time to move on.

*

It had always been part of my career plan to enter an emergency medicine program in the United States; they simply didn't exist in Canada at that time. Bob Scharf, the emergency medicine pioneer, and I had reached an agreement on this plan while I was working under his guidance as a medical student. While I was recovering from my accident, Bob didn't exactly press me to move into emergency medicine, but he was keen to remind me I had a career choice to make. He had located two possible options for me, both unfortunately far from home, where I would be "a stranger in a strange land." But both programs were developing into centres of excellence and were largely considered to be the leaders in the field. One was at the University of Cincinnati and the other at Los Angeles County/USC (LAC+USC) Medical Center, the USC program having full department status within a renowned medical school—University of Southern California.

I went to visit the people at University of Cincinnati one cold, grey, dreary day early in 1972. I was invited to interview for the Los Angeles program in April of that same year. What can I say? It was southern California—blue skies and coloured balloons and all the rest of it. LAC+USC Medical Center (rebranded in 2023 as Los Angeles General Medical Center) was a precious gem—or maybe just a diamond in the rough. The emergency department didn't turn away a soul, regardless of race, creed, colour, nationality, insurance status, or level of blood alcohol. This made LA County unusual if not unique among US hospitals. Our values were aligned and the weather was an additional attraction. That didn't mean I'd be accepted into the program, mind you. I later learned I was among sixty people applying for the last position in the program. Why was I accepted? That's still a bit of a mystery to me. I do know that US hospitals liked Canadian medical school graduates—especially those from Dalhousie—apparently because the Canucks spent so much more time in clinical practice, and less in book and classroom learning, than our US counterparts.

I wasn't about to question my good fortune, though, and I made my plans to head south by southwest while my colleagues in Neils Harbour planned a farewell party. There were cakes and scones and tea, of course, along with a few speeches I don't remember, no doubt singing my praises while bidding me a fond adieu. My departing gift was a treasure. Staff at the clinic had written to Charles Schulz—at that point my favourite author—and described how cartoons had helped restore me to brain health. Shultz responded by sending a signed copy of a cartoon showing Lucy lying on the ground at the base of Snoopy's doghouse. Snoopy, lying atop the doghouse in his characteristic pose— flat on his back, his nose in the air—doesn't budge to help Lucy. Lucy, being Lucy, demands an explanation. "Can't afford the malpractice insurance," Snoopy says. Or words to that effect. I'd quote the text verbatim, but I can't find the cartoon itself at the moment! (As I write this, I am moving my possessions into a new home for the final time in a long nomadic life. I'm hoping the cartoon is hiding in one of those boxes that I've dragged with me around the continent.)

In many ways, it was hard to say goodbye to the good people of Neils Harbour. They were dear people—my people—from close to my home. But it was time to move on. I packed up my Volvo station wagon and headed out on a six-day coast-to-coast drive to LA. The staff gathered on the steps of the Buchanan Memorial Hospital waving wildly, some tearful, and all admiring the large sign they had all signed beneath the huge letters—CALIFORNIA OR BUST! To Southern California, the land of the Beach Boys, the Mamas and the Papas, movie stars, and all the rest of it. Heck, even Charles Schulz lived in Santa Rosa. If I really harboured any delusion about looking him up, though, it was dead on arrival in LA.

"Mother County" and my career swallowed me whole on day one, and I wouldn't come out of the belly of the beast for another six years.

CHAPTER 5

HOLLYWOOD CALLING, 1972-1974

IT WAS QUITE A JOURNEY, THAT DRIVE FROM NEILS HARBOUR TO LOS ANGELES: TAKING THE big interstate highways all the way from the Atlantic to the Pacific; sleeping in my old Volvo at roadside rest areas like a character out of Kesey or Kerouac; moving from an all-white village of a few hundred people to a multicultural metropolis of a few million—from a place where problem drinkers quietly declined into isolated silence and sullen shame to the land of the celebrity overdose, where the stars flamed out on hot summer nights like meteors falling into earth's atmosphere.

In Neils Harbour, we treated a thousand or so patients *per year* at our small hospital's outpatient clinic. We saw many more in our family practice clinic in the village, typically for chronic conditions like hypertension or diabetes or cardiac failure. At the LAC+USC Medical Center, we treated up to a thousand patients *per day*, many of them victims of gunshot wounds, stabbings, or freeway crashes. (I had seen none of these in my years of undergraduate medical training or in general practice.)

I knew one thing for sure—I wasn't in Cape Breton anymore.

And I wasn't in Kansas either.

Instead, I was in a city that would consume my every moment until I departed six years later for a new position in Pittsburgh. I would spend my first three years in LA completing the emergency residency program at LAC+USC, and the last three on the streets and freeways of the city, where I would train LA's first generation of paramedics to treat the wounded where they lay. I also landed a third job in Los Angeles—one I didn't want but couldn't refuse. As the newest recruit to the emergency residency program in 1972, I ended up serving as the medical advisor to several TV shows, most notably *Emergency!*, which made heroes of LA firefighters as they responded to horrific freeway crashes and healthcare crises. This gig landed me with the unfortunate sobriquet "Doc Hollywood." It also, to my great surprise, taught me a great deal about winning friends, influencing people, and securing badly needed funding for healthcare services. (*Emergency!* became a cult classic, and in 2022, I was flown first-class to LA to attend a star-studded fiftieth reunion gala that packed a large auditorium to the rafters.[16])

Before I became counsel to the stars, however, I had to find the hospital itself. I managed to get a little lost at the end of my coast-to-coast odyssey. I had memorized the route to Los Angeles and its "County" hospital. I took the right exit off the I-10 (Soto Street) but at the bottom of the ramp I turned left, heading for a big white concrete building that sure as heck looked like LAC+USC (which I had seen only once before, during my interviews for the residency, a year or so previously). After climbing the imposing stairs of that concrete monolith, I found myself inside the East LA Sears building, and nervously asked an armed security guard for directions to the emergency department. He gently told me I was looking for the hospital everyone calls County and not (he was probably thinking) the ladies' lingerie department in which I appeared to have landed. A course correction northward took me to the hospital soon enough, but the story followed me around forever. (I made the mistake of telling the yarn to colleagues.)

I was like a kid in a candy shop when I started my residency at LA County. As a resident in emergency medicine, I was part of a pioneering effort to define best practices in modern emergency medical care in the US and beyond. My colleagues and I were not alone in this quest. I later realized that similar stories were unfolding at Cook County Hospital in Chicago, Bellevue Hospital in New York City, Charity in New Orleans, and several other city hospitals where health professionals gave their all to provide care to uninsured patients—many of them from Black, immigrant, or Hispanic communities. Our department's critical care receiving unit, known as C Booth, was shown in all its bloody glory in the 2013 documentary *Code Black*,[17] conceived and directed by Dr. Ryan McGarry, then a resident in the program I had completed forty years earlier. (A code Black was called when the emergency department was stretched beyond its normal limits, which was really saying something when waiting times for patients requiring non-urgent care were normally twelve hours or longer.) Stretchers in C Booth were crammed together; patients were surrounded by dozens of emergency staff; medical students in the famous teaching hospital watched the action, often by standing on chairs or counters and peering over the partitions separating C Booth from the rest of the department.

To a lay viewer, the C Booth scenes in McGarry's documentary look like pure chaos. Chests were cut open to massage hearts when this procedure was clinically indicated, often after a gun shot or stab wound. Defibrillators were primed and ready for action. Staff seem to buzz around like a swarm of bees disturbed from their nest. In fact, each professional in C Booth played an orchestral part in an extraordinary healthcare symphony. A senior resident or staff doctor picked up the baton as the conductor. A resident might be ready with the cardiac paddles, poised to jolt the patient back to life—or at least make an attempt. Attendants (often former military corpsmen trained on the job) could take charge of an Ambu bag, a hand-operated tool that ventilates the patient. Some staff would be in charge of administering IV fluids, others would stand by ready to deliver urgently needed medications—blood thinners, painkillers, or heart medications. Yet others might be dispatched to fetch a leg splint or medications or a suture kit.

As Dr. William "Billy" Mallon said in *Code Black*, C Booth was the place where "more people have died and more people have been saved than in any other square footage in the United States." (Mallon, a beloved and sharp-tongued physician from New Jersey, would become a legend in the annals of emergency medicine.) Earlier, I said I was like a kid in a candy shop in C Booth—because I learned so much from working there. Unlike some of the residents interviewed in *Code Black*, however, I was not thrilled by the prospect of someday running the show in C Booth, or by the inevitable adrenalin rush that accompanied the work. (For me, "terrified" would probably be a better descriptor than "thrilled.") What really bound me to one of America's biggest and best teaching hospitals was its values. When Mother County was opened in 1933, the inscription etched in stone above its entrance read, "The doctors of the staff give their services without charge in order that no citizens of the county shall be deprived of health or life for lack of such care and services." No insurance was required. This was the place for me, a place where, if my dad were transported through time and space, he could walk into the emergency department and have that severed thumb sewn back into place—just as he had in our tiny cottage hospital in Cape Breton in the early 1950s. So LA County felt to me, in some essential way, like home. It took all comers during the Depression years, when Hollywood actress Mary Pickford, a Canadian, dedicated an eight-ton cornerstone of the new building on State Street. Affiliated with the University of Southern California since 1885, the hospital—formally known as LAC+USC Medical Center—upholds the same values today that have defined it since the nineteenth century.

In other ways, of course, our tiny little hospital back home in Cape Breton was nothing like LA County. LA had so many stories, people, and experiences that could never have been part of my education had I spent my career in Nova Scotia. In May 1974, for instance, I joined colleagues on the roof of the hospital to watch a police shootout at 1466 East 54th Street, a few miles away. Members of the Symbionese Liberation Army (SLA) were holed up in a home at that address, and it was thought newspaper heiress Patty Hearst might be among them. (Hearst had been kidnapped by the organization a few months earlier and subsequently recruited into their ranks.) The standoff on East 54th was big news, covered live by the national TV networks. After one of the biggest shootouts in US police history, with an estimated nine thousand shots fired, the standoff ended when the home caught fire. Patty Hearst was not among the SLA members found at the scene; she had watched the drama unfold on television. She would later be convicted of bank robbery and ended up serving two years of a seven-year jail sentence before President Jimmy Carter commuted her sentence. Back at the hospital on that fateful night, we retreated from our rooftop vantage point, anticipating ambulances to race casualties to our emergency department. It didn't happen. All six members of the SLA holed up in the home had died, most of them from smoke inhalation. There were no casualties or serious injuries among the hundreds of police officers and FBI agents on the scene.

By the time of the shootout, I had been in LA for about eighteen months, but I still couldn't quite believe what I was watching from the rooftop. Nothing in my past experience as a physician—or in my wider life in Nova Scotia—had prepared me for a night like that. In addition, nothing had prepared me for the long row of phone booths, built into the wall along the corridor just outside our department, that indigent people eventually transformed into sleeping quarters. Nothing prepared me for cutting open a patient's chest to apply open-heart massage, sometimes, in the urgency of the moment, forgetting to don protective gloves. Nothing prepared me for a rotation, as a young resident in the program, that took me from the primary care unit of the emergency department—where I might have to treat a cold—to the minor trauma unit where a broken leg might be casted; to a unit where we treated ambulatory patients with non-complex medical problems; to the general medicine service of the hospital, and to the jail ward in the hospital, where I came face-to-face with (among others) the infamous cult leader Charles Manson, whose followers had broken into actress Sharon Tate's home in 1969, killing her and four others.

The jail ward was a world unto itself. Operated by the LA County Department of Corrections and staffed by Corrections Service employees, it seemed to live by its own rules. We suspected some of the jail guards didn't operate to the highest ethical standards, and we were only slightly surprised that patients occasionally attempted to escape the ward by throwing themselves down the laundry chute. The ward was on the thirteenth floor of the hospital, a long way from the laundry room in one of the three sub-basements of the facility. During my time at LAC+USC, rumour had it that at least three prisoners took the desperate plunge. Two were said to have died, while one survived after landing in a huge pile of laundry.

To say the least, these incidents were suspicious. To begin with, everything on the ward was supposed to be locked, including the laundry chute door. In theory, there was only one way to leave the ward, via an elevator that was well secured behind several locks—an elevator protected by an armed guard. An internal inquiry convened to review the laundry chute deaths uncovered widespread corruption. Not only could prisoners take their slim chances in the laundry chute; they could also gain access to drugs—brought in by family members with the help of prison staff who were all too eager to supplement their income by taking bribes from the suppliers or prisoners. The findings of the hospital inquiry were kept hush-hush, though the *Los Angeles Times* later referred to one of the laundry chute divers in a story published in 2006.[18] The poor soul described in the *Times* story escaped the fall with only a broken leg and then managed to trace an agonizing route through the hospital's labyrinth of underground tunnels. He did make his way to the street, only to be picked up there by police.

Charles Manson never threw himself down the laundry chute from the jail ward, but he was occasionally sent to the "the County" when he went off his meds—to use the colloquial phrase. Several of us suspected his medications were manipulated by prison staff who wanted to get him out of their hair for a few days. Our job was to titrate his medications and send him back to prison. (He was housed in several different prisons until he died in 2017 at the ripe old age of eighty-three.) I only recall treating him once—for an infection of some sort, I believe—but his reputation certainly preceded him, and I certainly recall his vacant-eyed stare. Whether that faraway look was a product of his illness or his medications or my own apprehension—or all three—I cannot really say.

It says something about our obsession with celebrity culture that I knew more about Charles Manson than I did about the formidable Margaret McCarron before I met both on the LAC+USC jail ward. Dr. McCarron, who died in 2007 at the age of seventy-nine, educated thousands of physicians and pharmacists over a forty-two–year period at LAC+USC, thirty-five of them as the hospital's Associate Medical Director. I first knew her as a straight-talking Illinois native who acted and sounded confident enough to survive, if not thrive, on what was—from the point of view of doctor–patient relationships, at least—the toughest ward to practise medicine on at Mother County. McCarron learned lessons that only a jail ward could teach—what kind of small bags were best used to transport illegal drugs inside inmate bellies, how street narcotics could interact (often dangerously) with other medications, and how to recognize and treat bowel obstructions caused by what came to be called body-packing—the ingestion of hard drugs in small bags that sometimes led to bowel obstruction in the unfortunate "packer." She offered her often-mocked patients on the jail ward compassionate care and demanded they be treated with the respect all patients deserve, whether they were handcuffed to their hospital beds or not. A pioneer in educating students about how to treat people with AIDS at a time when they were ostracized, her obituary in the *LA Times* lauds her as an innovator whose "teaching of pharmacy practice changed…pharmacy training into what it is today, known as Clinical Pharmacy." It's a measure of her teaching excellence that McCarron quickly recognized me as a fish out of water at LAC+USC. I was shocked by what I saw on the jail ward—a fact I tried to hide. She saw through it immediately and took me under her wing. She somehow knew where I was from and what I was like. She was the right kind of mentor for me at the right time, as I tried to navigate a strange new world in LA.

As I progressed in the three-year residency program at LAC+USC, I spent more and more time treating seriously injured or ill patients in C Booth of the emergency department itself. In the first year of my residency, C Booth functioned largely as a triage unit—shuffling patients off to appropriate wards upstairs. Critically ill or injured patients arriving in C Booth were quickly assessed, then expedited "upstairs" after a small red blanket was thrown on the stretcher to indicate that their problem was urgent. "Red blanket" became a noun, a verb, and an adjective in our lexicon: "We have a red blanket coming in by ambulance"; "Red blanket this patient upstairs"; "That red-blanket patient was definitely a challenge"—these phases were in everyday use. In C Booth, medical teams treated those most at risk of imminent death.

It's crucial to understand that the LAC+USC was (and is) surrounded by African American, Latino, and Asian neighbourhoods in under-resourced communities that gathered together under the "Friday night lights" of local high school football matches. In the trenches of the department, the emergency care team dubbed the Friday evening football events "Friday night fights"—a reflection of the parade of the walking wounded and seriously injured who came or were transported from high school football stadiums to our hospital. Bullet and knife wounds were not unusual, and family members and friends of the victims would invariably show up at the hospital en masse to watch and pray over their loved ones. It fell to the staff doctors to inform family members when a patient had left this world for a better one. Loved ones were invited to vacate the always-crowded waiting room for a smaller private room in which the bad news was communicated. To understand how important this protocol was, readers have to understand what was going on in the waiting room on football Friday nights. Rival gang members, along with family members and friends of both patients, waited in vigilant—and sometime vigilante-style—attendance while the victims of violence were treated.

On one occasion, a surgical resident unfamiliar with the emergency department protocol broke the bad news of a patient's death in the middle of the waiting room itself. Everyone, of course, was listening. You can imagine what happened next. The dead boy's gang members were there, and so were members of the rival gang who had shot him. Guns were drawn and fired in the crowded waiting room as the poor kid's brothers-in-arms sought to avenge his death. Bullets were flying. I recall the evening with good reason—I was in C Booth (not far from the waiting area) when the gunfire burst out. I was "bagging" a patient—using a bag valve mask (BVM) to pump oxygen into the lungs of a victim of the Friday night fights. Fearful that stray ammunition might be headed my way, I crouched with a nurse and orderly under the stretcher with my arm curled over the mattress and my hand still compressing the bag. How long this lasted remains unclear to me, but in the mayhem of the moment, despite our attempts at resuscitation, the lad was dead even before the gunfire ceased. I spent much of the remainder of my shift searching for his relatives before giving up and crawling back to bed in the nearby intern quarters. I never did find the relatives.

The realization that I was in a different culture—and world—in Los Angeles often struck with force at Mother County. Many, if not most, of our patients spoke Spanish and their culture was, to say the least, unfamiliar to me. An incident early on in my residency bears witness to how unfamiliar it was. I vividly recall the death of a young Latino boy from gang warfare; indeed, it has never left me. After we had done our best, yet failed to save him, I found his loved ones in the waiting room, and escorted his large entourage—mother, grandmother, and I don't know who else—to a small out-of-the-way office to break the news. I was very direct in my language—we always said the patient had "died," not that he had "passed away" or "left this earth" or "gone to a better place." If the tragic message was to sink in, plain, simple, monosyllabic English would be required. Unfortunately, in this, as in many other cases, plain Spanish would have worked better. I couldn't speak the family's language, and they didn't understand mine. When I finally got through to the boy's mother, she let out a loud wail and fell against me, clutching onto me in the process. Her mother then fell against her, and I was soon pinned to the floor under a heap of loudly grieving relatives. As a Calvinist boy from a culture where the stoically bereaved were comforted by four muttered words—"sorry for your loss"—this was a shocking experience. But it was one I learned to manage, and manage well, I hope. Like most Canadians, I don't tend to see my life as a series of highlight reels, but I can say that one of my proudest moments came during an exit interview I conducted once with a resident at Mother County. Almost in tears, she surprised me by saying she decided to choose emergency medicine as a career after watching me talk with family members quietly and compassionately about the death of a loved one.

Through the Friday night fights, through my work on the prison and medical wards, and through the various tiers of the emergency department, I learned a heck of a lot about my chosen specialty—and myself—during my three-year residency at LAC+USC Medical Center. Robert (Bob) Dailey, the director of the emergency medicine residency program, was hands-down my most important mentor. Dailey, whom I grew to consider a good friend, selected me for the residency program from among a crowded field of applicants and even put me up in his apartment when I was interviewed for the position. Dailey was an early pioneer in this new area of emergency medicine and a brilliant teacher—a standout in a field largely populated by burnouts. In the early 1970s, the emergency departments of hospitals were often a refuge of last resort for docs with addiction problems or other issues. It's never been entirely clear to me why Dailey chose me for the residency program. (It is clear that Dailey, McCarron, and my experiences in the trenches were the best teachers during my residency program at Mother County.) He might have known that Dalhousie's medical school sent docs into the world with lots of clinical experience due to our baptism of fire rotating through various specialities in the last year of the program. I also suspect I got a quiet nod from Dr. John "Jack" Bethune. Like me, Bethune was a Nova Scotian, an Acadia grad, and a Dalhousie medical school grad. His storied career took him to Harvard and London before he left his professorship at Dal to take a position in 1961 at LAC+USC. In 1972, the same year I moved to LA, Bethune was named chair of the department of medicine at USC, and chief of medicine at the hospital. Dailey might well have consulted Bethune about my application.

While Dailey taught me a lot about being a physician, my work as a consultant to Hollywood television shows offered a very different kind of education. (Initially, I only gave a few hours of my time to this job each week, but the demands it made on me seemed to grow significantly over time. I continued to do the work after finishing my residency program, but I knew I had to ease out of it after taking on a job training paramedics.) It was through my Doc Hollywood role that I really started to learn about the politics of healthcare. The American Medical Association—then as now a powerful lobby group—played a role as watchdog and medical censor on all network shows. All doctors were to be portrayed as angelic, and no patient was to die. Break the rules and you wouldn't get advisory help from young residents like me. Nor would you get affordable access to the medical equipment or healthcare settings that gave the shows at least a thin veneer of authenticity. For the AMA, this was all about managing the message and the profile of the profession. If doctors were seen to be kindly healers—a bit closer to Christ than mere mortals—legislators in state houses and Washington would take notice when the AMA lobbied on its members' behalf.

How did I end up enmeshed in this odd Holly-world? Not long after I landed in LA, I was persuaded to act as a consultant to some network television shows including *Marcus Welby, M.D.*, but more extensively with the NBC series *Emergency!*, which was broadcast for seven years starting in 1972. Though I was a reluctant and unpaid recruit, my work with the show earned me an enduring amount of modest fame. The show featured the adventures of Squad 51, a Paramedic rescue service created inside the LA County Fire Department's rescue units. This was high-adventure docudrama featuring car crashes and heroic, improbably successful efforts to revive nearly dead victims. I served as script reviewer and medical advisor. I suggested medically reasonable scenarios for writers, took phone calls from producers, made sure the right medical equipment got delivered to the film sets, and generally made a nuisance of myself by insisting the crew and cast get the medical bits right. (On-set paramedics were the *real* guardians of medical accuracy—such as it was in the early days of the show.) To be honest, the show captured the public's imagination more than it did my own. (Confession here: I have never owned a television and never watched a full episode of the show. I did see some of the dailies—video of scenes shot that day—when I was on the set.)

If the show could be described as melodrama, the behind-the-scenes action on the set would more accurately be characterized as soap opera. Consider the cast and crew for a moment: The co-producer and creator was Jack Webb, of *Dragnet* fame. The cast included Webb's ex-wife, the torch singer Julie London, who was said to have landed the role of nurse Dixie McCall as part of the terms of her divorce settlement with Webb. Turns out London was then singing duets with another musician—her new husband Bobby Troup: singer, pianist, and composer Bobby Troup, who wrote "Route 66." Incredibly, he was also cast in the show as Dr. Joe Early. Robert (Bob) Cinader, Webb's co-producer, was a classic cigar-chomping, foul-mouthed New Yorker. Cinader, who worked with Webb on *Dragnet*, was really the brains behind the show—he came up with the concept in the first place. (He became fully schooled in the developing paramedic system in Southern California and actually had several appointments to Emergency Services Commissions and advisory boards. The fire station used on the show was renamed the Robert A. Cinader Fire Station after he died in 1982.) Robert Fuller played Dr. Kelly Brackett, whose character was said to be modelled after me. (That was embarrassing for both of us.) In short, the set was one volatile mix of personalities. You had Julie London. You had her ex-husband. You had her new husband. You had Bob Cinader. It was ripe for spontaneous combustion.

Like politics, show business makes for strange bedfellows. I became a close friend to Cinader, who was smart and savvy and sophisticated—and kind—under that gruff exterior. Earlier in his career, he had run the publications division at the United Nations. Despite my early distaste for my role in what I thought was a not-so-academic, even frivolous treatment of the serious stuff of human health and suffering, I felt myself changing over time. I began to realize how influential the show proved to be in fostering public awareness of the importance of immediate care of illness and injury. In addition, I became a close friend of several members of the cast and crew—certainly with Bob Cinader, but also with Kevin Tighe and Randy Mantooth, who played the Squad 51 paramedics on the show. One of my "duties" as the show developed was to accompany Kevin or Randy to medical conferences and meetings and field any "medical" questions or issues that might come up. For Julie London, I was sometimes a shoulder to cry on. I was surprised that her first call was to me the day her mother, vaudeville veteran Josephine Peck, died in 1976. After that loss, we talked occasionally rather than frequently, and after that I left LA within a couple of years and lost touch with her. Alas, I often played the role of the "shoulder to cry on" in my relationships with women, although I sometimes yearned for more—a wife, a family, kids, a house in the burbs. By 1974, though, my marriage to medicine had been shown to be tested and true. In my three years in the residency program, I'd barely had time to sleep in my monk's cell in the residents' dorm, let alone pursue a relationship with a colleague, a Hollywood actress, or even a waitress awaiting her big chance.

I gradually came to realize, during my LA years and afterward, that my snooty attitude about the Doc Hollywood role was ill-advised and superficial. As a skinny kid from Canada who'd landed a residency in emergency medicine, I was no one to the powers-that-were in LA. As medical advisor to major TV shows, I was hardly a glittering star in the Hollywood firmament, but I was only a few light years away from the heavenly bodies. My job as reluctant counsel-to-the-stars opened doors for me. The people at the LA County and LA city fire departments, key players in the ambulance response systems, knew me or knew about me. It also turned out that *Emergency!* itself fed a public demand for improved emergency healthcare services.

In an odd way, my work in TV taught me something about the effectiveness of my boss at LAC+USC, Dr. Gail Anderson. Anderson, who died in 2014 at the age of eighty-eight, was named as the first chair of the department of emergency medicine in 1971. Indeed, he was the first chair of an academic department of emergency medicine anywhere in the US, where the speciality wouldn't be officially recognized until 1978. We residents were frankly befuddled by our boss's appointment. He was trained as a gynecologist and obstetrician and had headed the hospital's ob/gyn department since 1958. Why put him in charge of the emergency department? Well, we had it all wrong. To begin with, Anderson had served as a miliary corpsman in the Second World War, a role in which he had treated wounded soldiers. More importantly, he was a mover and shaker and networker of the first rank. A big, good-looking man with an imposing manner—always dressed in a starched white lab coat—Anderson commanded respect the minute he walked into a room. (His imperious very-Southern drawl also played its part in creating a commanding presence.) Anderson's colleagues say he quickly moved to consolidate emergency medicine as a speciality at the hospital, and to secure the funding to do the job right.[19] More importantly, he finessed the creation of the specialty department in the university—probably the most important of his achievements. That brought opportunities for research, recruitment of quality staff, and publicity; all these are, of course, the basis of power—and they attract the top tier of trainees from the medical schools in the US and beyond. I was slow to understand just how crucial Anderson was to the delivery of quality care. He accomplished this not through clinical teaching or by example, but through his superb command of hospital and healthcare politics. Just as my experience as Doc Hollywood showed me that public sentiment can drive health policy, Gail Anderson's example was proof positive that the delivery of better care at the stretcher or hospital bed was enabled by internal champions who knew how to "work the system." This was one valuable lesson I would try to put to good use in my future career in medical and civilian politics.

Mind you, we still had some way to go—both at the hospital and in the streets. The sad truth was that the paramedics on the TV show delivered better care than most residents of the county and city of LA received. On *Emergency!* few, if any, patients died from cardiac arrest or major trauma—thanks in part to the oversight of the AMA. In the streets of LA, and before the emergency medical services program was widespread, hardly anyone survived a cardiac arrest in the street. That didn't improve much, even in the first few years after the program began, because we had no concept that other factors were involved—public CPR education, 911 systems—all essential elements in the "chain of survival."

The root cause of this tragic record was, in the beginning, a legacy system that was cumbersome and time-consuming. To begin with, few first responders—dispatched from either the fire departments or the funeral homes—were well trained. They could put on bandages, and most were trained to perform cardiopulmonary resuscitation (CPR), but that was it. If a patient at the roadside or in the home was in ventricular fibrillation, in the early months of the EMS program, the responding paramedic squad had to drive to the one participating hospital, fetch the coronary unit nurse from the upper floor of the hospital, and drive her to the scene where the patient could be "legally" defibrillated. Very few patients survived. *Emergency!* drove public demand for better emergency healthcare response, though, and attracted a new generation of paramedics to the field.

In short, the demand for better-trained paramedics and better emergency healthcare was well-seeded and well-fertilized by the time I finished my residency program in 1974. The timing, for me, was pure serendipity. Within a year of finishing my residency, I was juggling more balls than a circus clown. I was appointed director of pre-hospital care programs for the department of emergency medicine at LAC+USC as well as director of the Paramedic Training Institute (PTI) for the county, and made an assistant professor at USC's department of emergency medicine. I was also struggling to keep my promise to serve as an advisor to *Emergency!* and other doc shows.

In all these roles save the last one, I had a single mission—I had to make life imitate art. I had to bring Hollywood-style emergency care standards into the real world. I would strive, for the next four years, to turn illusion into reality.

CHAPTER 6

THE TOASTER WARS AND OTHER LESSONS IN LA POLITICS, 1974-1978

LAC+USC ALWAYS SEEMED TO BE IN A STATE OF FLUX OR CHAOS OR CRISIS. AND ALL THREE hit me at once as I was shifting from my residency program to my new job in paramedic training. Bob Dailey, the man who plucked me out of Cape Breton Island and plunked me down in central LA, left town in 1974 for a new job as director of the emergency department at Valley Medical Center in Fresno, California. His departure dealt a body blow to the residents left behind. We were largely self-taught in the emergency residency program at County, and our attending physicians often seemed to be missing in action. Dailey was the exception. He did his best to educate us in the emerging art (and science) of emergency medicine. As one of my fellow residents later put it, "our group was pissed [about Dailey's departure] because he *was* the residency."[20]

Dailey offered to take me with him to central California to work with him in a senior position at the hospital in Fresno. His offer surprises me less today than it did in 1974. Though I was yet to finish my residency, emergency medicine was still a burgeoning field, and I was an educable physician who had undergone a baptism of fire in my chosen field. In short, I was a live body to throw into the trenches. In my mind, however, my long-term destination was not the west coast of America but the east coast of Canada, where I hoped to someday join forces with my old mentor Bob Scharf from Dalhousie University. Sadly, that goal was out of reach—emergency medicine would not be recognized as a speciality in Canada until 1980, so I had no job in my specialty to return to in my homeland.

Scharf would have been a perfect recruit to replace Dailey in LA, though I doubted he'd be willing to say farewell to Nova Scotia.

We were a tight, hard-working group, and when we discussed the departure of Dailey from our midst, we all agreed it would be wise to see if Bob Scharf might join us in LA as the new director of the LAC+USC residency program. No one was better qualified than the man who had sent me into the streets of Halifax with ambulance attendants a few years previously. I never for a moment thought Scharf and his wife Betty, a native Nova Scotian with deep ties to the province, would migrate west to take a position at LAC+USC, but I made the call to him anyway. I was gobsmacked when he said he would consider an offer. The job was his to take if he wanted it, and it turned out he did. Next day, he called back to say he and Betty would move west to LA.

Sadly, I would see less of Scharf in LA than I anticipated. I continued to work as an attending physician at the County emergency department after I finished my residency, so our paths occasionally crossed. But more and more of my time was taken up with the paramedic training program, and less and less of it with the hospital or the set of *Emergency!* No wonder—my job as the director of the Paramedic Training Institute for the county was a crash course in the complicated world of LA politics.

Talk about competing agendas. The fire departments for LA County and the City of Los Angeles, both players in emergency response services, were bitter rivals. Add to this toxic brew the funeral homes, which ran private for-profit ambulance services. The funeral-home model of care was at least a simple one: get the patients to hospital and hope they don't die in the meantime. In essence, the vehicles used were taxicabs with stretchers in the back, or more accurately hearses equipped either with stretchers for one final trip to a hospital or coffins for one final trip to a cemetery. Early on, personnel were trained to no recognized standards, though the more progressive homes took steps to provide better care. Overall, from the point of view of quality of medical care, the funeral homes were certainly not hitting the mark. The funeral home operators earned top grades as lobbyists, however. They maintained close ties with business organizations and politicians and leveraged those relationships to the hilt. Add to that the half-dozen or so hospitals involved in emergency medicine; the cardiac nurses providing training to some first responders; and the medical schools at USC and UCLA, and you'll start to get a sense of the murky waters I was trying to navigate.

And then, to trump them all, there was the LA County Board of Supervisors, an elected body with both executive and legislative responsibilities inside what has been called "the largest and most complex county government in the entire United States."[21] I'll venture a little further here and try to describe the rabbit warren of LA politics. The City of LA, with its own mayor and councillors, is only one of several municipalities operating under the umbrella government of the County of Los Angeles, which was created by the state legislature in 1852. Jurisdictional boundaries between city and county governments were sometimes vague, and sometimes guarded by fierce partisans on both sides—as was the case with the LA County and city fire departments. (In the greater LA area, there were about forty-nine fire departments.) My job involved earning some measure of co-operation from the LA County and city departments—a daunting task, as I would soon discover. As the guy managing paramedic training, I struggled to work the system at the distinct LA nexus where politics, governance, and a bewildering ground of stakeholders overlapped—that is, before the elected County Board of Supervisors and various subcommittees, which set budgets and approved spending.

Nothing better illustrates the challenges of dealing with that august body than the story of the "toaster wars." I got myself onto the agenda of a subcommittee of the county board, one made up largely of fire chiefs and politicians. My goal was replacing the antiquated suction units then used by emergency responders in the department(s). Frankly, you couldn't suck spit through the suction equipment they were then using. I had a proposal ready to go. I came armed with flow rates and other technical data, along with a proposal to buy new state-of-the-art suction units manufactured by the Norwegian firm Laerdal Medical, a leading global supplier of emergency medical devices. I wasn't too alarmed when the LA County fire chief got to present his own proposal first—he requested deluxe new toasters for his fire stations, what I called "six-seaters" to toast half a dozen slices of bread at once. (Talk about state-of-the-art!) I was bemused rather than alarmed when the $80,000 toaster purchase was approved in a few minutes. Bemusement turned to bewilderment when the meeting suddenly closed. I hadn't even had a chance to make my case to the committee. How could new toasters possibly be more important than life-saving medical equipment? There was no good answer to that question. All I knew was that the six-seaters carried the day. That meeting represented a loss of innocence for this miner's son from Sydney Mines. Fortunately, paramedics and first responders are tinkerers and problem-solvers by nature, and we managed to jury-rig adequate suction equipment in most of our emergency response vehicles for what I hoped would be the short term until new equipment arrived.

I was also to meet another creative tinkerer during my early years in LA. Geoffrey Garth first showed up in my life at an Emergency Medical Services conference in San Diego at which I had taken the podium to complain about the sorry state of the equipment we were forced to use in our paramedic practice. Most of the gear—cumbersome steel oxygen cylinders, heavy defibrillators, underpowered suction equipment—was designed for use in hospitals or other clinical settings.

It wasn't suited to emergency response at freeway crashes or accidents in the home or on the beach—places where emergency medical equipment often had to be hauled by hand.

Geoff had been attending a toy convention of some sort in the same conference complex at which I spoke, and he showed up at my event out of sheer boredom. The inappropriate use of soft cervical collars must have been one of my pet peeves that day, because at the end of my talk, Geoff—then a designer at Mattel toys—came up and told me he could design a cervical collar that would keep a patient's head in place and the cervical spine stable. We were then using soft orthopedic collars, usually borrowed from a friendly hospital, and the best you could say for them was that they kept a patient comfortable while they were on the way to becoming quadriplegic.

I told Geoff to get back to me if he designed a hard plastic cervical collar that would work. I was impressed that he seemed to know what he was talking about despite having no medical training, but I figured that was the last I'd ever see of him. He seemed like a cool and creative California surfer dude, and I suspected toy design would not captivate him for his whole career. Well, I was right about the cool and creative elements of Geoff's character, but it turned out he also had an absolute genius for design—and for entrepreneurship. A few months after the San Diego event, he showed up at my office in LA with several hard plastic cervical collars in various sizes—including some designed for children.

Within a few years, Geoff had formed his own medical company, California Medical Products, and he was well on his way to becoming very successful indeed based on his business savvy and creative flair as a designer. We became close friends and kept in touch for decades. He would later invite me to go with him around the world as he introduced his medical devices while I met with emergency personnel, armed with my tray of slides and ready to preach the gospel of better emergency care in the streets—treating people where they lie. In addition, I had a few other ideas about better "medical mousetraps" I knew might interest him. His role was to show off his medical devices and introduce me. I was happy to endorse his company because he really had built a number of better mousetraps—so to speak—when it came to emergency medical equipment.

I wish I could say my tussle to obtain quality suction units was my only struggle as I attempted to support and improve the paramedic training program. Far from it. So far from it, in fact, that when I look back at those years, I wonder how I survived. To improve pre-hospital emergency care in LA, I had to tread on a lot of the toes of people who quickly decided that disliking me personally was their best option. The private ambulance operators weren't about to welcome reform quietly, nor did many of them want to spend extra money to train first responders. A deal was finally struck that teamed ambulance operators with the fire departments in LA County. (The City of LA had its own ambulances.) The first responders from the fire stations would treat patients at the scene, and then call the private ambulances—dubbed "the privates" by the medics—to transport patients. The paramedics would have to squeeze into the back of the privately owned ambulances to get patients to the hospital. The system was cumbersome, inefficient, and driven by the needs of stakeholders with little understanding of pre-hospital care. The private ambulance operators, a powerful political lobby, wanted a piece of the action. Politicians wanted to please their campaign donors—those same operators. There was no ill intent in any of this, but you'd never design a system like this to benefit patients first.

I also worked closely with the coronary care nurses who tradition-ally had trained paramedics from the fire departments. This group of nurses—about twenty of them in all—were well versed in one aspect of emergency healthcare: coronary care, of course. And paramedics were trained to very high standards indeed in coronary care. The challenge was that only about 10 percent of emergency calls were related to a cardiac event. Broken limbs, cuts, gunshot wounds—paramedics had to help patients suffering from all of these problems, and sometimes all of them at once. I broadened the curriculum for paramedics and brought in additional instructors with expertise in a wide variety of fields. Fortunately, the nurses involved in the program took their duty of care seriously and understood the need to diversify the curriculum.

I was also fortunate to work with the paramedics from the fire stations, many of whom had served as medics or soldiers in the Vietnam War. I spent a lot of time with them in the streets of LA, so much so that I can still find my way around the big city more easily than I can in little Halifax, the provincial capital of my home province of Nova Scotia. Their experience in the field of war prepared them to staunch bleeds on the streets of the city. They performed their tasks with more skill and savvy than most medical practitioners, and I formed a quick bond with them by respecting their work. Their experience in battle had conditioned them to act quickly in an emergency, and in doing so to save lives and limbs. Working closely with paramedics, I recognized that some of them were experiencing mental health problems of their own. I also knew the old remedies (a stiff upper lip and a bottle of booze) for what we now call post-traumatic stress disorder were counterproductive at best.

Looking back, I see that the distressing "toaster wars" meeting was my initiation into LA politics—and politics in general. It took a couple of years to finally get the new suction units, by the way. In the meantime, I learned, through my battle with funeral home operators, fire chiefs, politicians, and old-school firefighters themselves that I was fighting the toughest opponent of all in medicine—the status quo. Hardly anyone seemed to like change, even within a system that badly needed it.

Fortunately, not all the news was bad, and while the micro-politics in LA posed deadly risks to emergency patients, national politics and global trends in healthcare were working in our favour. Indeed, reforms in civilian trauma care can be traced both nationally and internationally to the mid-1960s. In 1966, the National Academy of Sciences of the United States, an obscure group which advised Congress, teamed up with the US National Research Council to publish an explosive report on traumatic injury and death. Even its title—*Accidental Death and Disability: The Neglected Disease of Modern Society*[22]—minced no words. It reported more than 100,000 US deaths from highway crashes and other traumatic events in 1965. The report found that emergency departments were inadequate, attending physicians were woefully untrained, and ambulance and helicopter transport systems needed to be reorganized. The NAC–NRC story was a hot item in the media for a short time, but the authors left it cooking on the stove by distributing thousands of copies to state and federal legislators across the US. The issue simmered slowly until 1973, when Congress passed the Emergency Medical Services (EMS) Act. (Yes, the gestation period in politics is often long enough to put the elephant to shame—a reality I was to face after I was later named health minister in Nova Scotia in 1993.) The act put standards in place for emergency care, and funds were allocated to build out regional EMS systems and train emergency healthcare professionals. Virtually no one tells the story of the final passage of the EMS Act,[23] by the way, without mentioning the influence of *Emergency!* on members of Congress—further proof of the fact that infotainment trumps information when it comes to influencing public opinion and politicians.

American commentators tend to see their nation as the birthplace of modern emergency medicine practices, and it is true that the practice evolved with astonishing speed in the US throughout the 1970s. But if you're looking for the real birthplace of modern EMS, you have to cast an eye on the innovative Irish. Two figures emerge as EMS leaders in the creation of what became known as the Belfast Flying Squad, the world's first mobile coronary care unit. One was Frank Pantridge (1916–2004), a native of County Down who volunteered for the British Army after finishing medical school. Pantridge was sent to serve in Singapore just before it was captured by the Japanese, who put the tough Ulsterman in a POW camp for the rest of the war. He survived the internment despite all odds, and happily returned to (as he put it) "breathe the free air of County Down."[24] Pantridge's colleague, John Geddes, a graduate of Queen's University of Belfast, was twenty years younger than Pantridge and both more studious and more diplomatic. (Pantridge was infamously irascible. He would often tell slow-learning medical students under his charge to "get out of [their] coma." Geddes and Pantridge knew from the research record that most people experiencing a heart attack (myocardial infarction) died within an hour of the incident and away from hospital. Treating the minority of patients who made it to hospital after a heart attack was reaching only the tip of the iceberg, Pantridge said.[25]

This was the fundamental insight on which the Belfast Flying Squad was set loose in the streets of Belfast on New Year's Day 1966. This was not a sleek or a slick operation. Geddes and Pantridge commandeered a dilapidated ambulance for the job and staffed it with a physician-led team of nurses, medical students, and drivers. The equipment included a 75-kilogram defibrillator, so the medical team had to be both skilled and strong. (Pantridge, Geddes, and electrical engineer Alfred Mawhinney would later design a 3.5-kilogram model known as the Pantridge defibrillator.) The story of the Flying Squad has an enduring place in EMS history because the team saved lives in the streets on Belfast. This news (gradually) made its way to America and around the world after Pantridge and Geddes published their landmark paper, "A Mobile Intensive-Care Unit in the Management of Myocardial Infarction"[26] in the *Lancet* in August 1967. The authors reported that ten patients were resuscitated outside of hospital, and five were still "alive and well" at the time of publication. The authors state, modestly, "Thus it has been shown perhaps for the first time that the correction of cardiac arrest outside hospital is a practicable proposition."

South of the Irish border, in the Republic of Ireland, a Dublin cardiac care team was quick to adapt the Belfast model. Instead of a flying squad, the Dubliners in essence created the first generation of real paramedics, who were freed up to go flying on their own. That is, they could defibrillate and resuscitate patients in the field without being directly supervised by senior medical personnel—that is, by doctors or cardiac-care nurses. These ambulance teams—two to a vehicle—were trained extensively in cardiopulmonary resuscitation, the operation of defibrillators, reading EKGs, and every other element of care that cardiac nurses then learned. The Dublin story is fully outlined in "Prehospital Coronary Care Service," published in the July 1971 edition of the *British Medical Journal.* The coronary care ambulance system, run by the Irish Heart Foundation, was remarkably efficient and effective, the authors concluded. Response times were remarkable; seventeen or twenty patients were successfully defibrillated, and no patients died in an ambulance during the time period covered by the report. Perhaps more significantly, doctors—there was a shortage of physicians in Dublin at the time—were left to do work more suited to their skills. "In light of this experience the routine employment of doctors may be unnecessary and involve an uneconomical use of their skills." The authors went on to say the Dublin model of emergency coronary care "is the best system for most urban areas using a hospital rota system."[27]

US cities adopted the Irish models quickly enough, with Seattle leading the way in terms of putting trained paramedic teams in place to administer coronary care procedures. In LA, the need for emergency care reform was urgent. The weaknesses in the City of Los Angeles ambulance system were brutally exposed following the assassination of Robert Kennedy at the Ambassador Hotel in June 1968. Suffering from a serious brain injury from a gunshot wound, RFK was thrown onto a stretcher and taken to the LA Receiving Hospital, located in the middle of the city. The emergency department often looked after street people and others from the neighbourhood, and it had neither the facilities nor the staff to treat someone in RFK's condition. Kennedy was then taken to Good Samaritan Hospital, where he would finally be pronounced dead about twenty-six hours after he had been shot. (His injuries were severe enough that he likely would have died regardless of the treatment he received.)

Good Samaritan Hospital was often described in media reports as an excellent centre for neurological and neurosurgical care. Fair enough. Its medical teams were experienced in the treatment of non-traumatic brain injuries or illnesses. But patients with gunshot wounds—often from marginalized communities—would routinely be turned away from the Good Samaritan because they didn't carry health insurance. If you needed treatment for gunshot wounds to the head, or anyplace else, LAC+USC was the place to go. There, the medical teams and neurosurgeons dealt with traumatic injuries daily. This fact was largely lost in the uproar following RFK's assassination. What was clear was the fact that the LA ambulance system was in sad shape. A grand jury was convened to investigate the emergency services response after RFK's death. The City of LA then made a wise, if belated, decision to assign EMS first responders to every fire station and initiated a paramedic training program beginning with the original program at Harbour General. My boss, Gail Anderson, his political antennae as finely tuned as ever, welcomed the invitation to expand the program at LAC+USC. I was recruited to run it in 1974.

If the micro-politics of funeral homes and fire departments conspired against my success in my new job, I quickly realized that the macro-politics were in my favour. Two years after RFK's assassination, on July 15, 1970, Governor Ronald Reagan signed a law (the Wedworth-Townsend Paramedic Act), which allowed trained mobile intensive-care paramedics to deliver care at the scene rather than just take them to hospital. Crucially, it allowed paramedics to puncture the skin (administer medication), defibrillate heart patients, and perform other treatments at the scene or on the way to hospital. It also exempted medical staff from legal liability related to paramedic care administered in good faith. Reagan was reluctant to sign the bill into law—the first state paramedic law in the nation—over the objections of nurses and doctors. He only did so after the act was amended, sensibly, to allow ambulances to cross municipal lines within LA County. (Reagan's father, Jack, had died from a heart attack in 1941 after a City of LA ambulance had followed the rules—stopping at the border of the city rather than entering the exclusive enclave where Jack lived.[28]) The act was first drafted by a sort of legislative odd couple, LA County Supervisor Kenneth Hahn and Dr. Walter Graf, a legendary pioneer in the practice of emergency medicine. (Graf died in 2015 at the age of ninety-eight.) Within a month of the passage of the act, Graf and his colleague Dr. Michael Criley set up the first formal paramedic training program in the state. (Informally, they had started training paramedics in pre-hospital coronary care earlier in 1970.)

As for Kenneth Hahn, he was a politician of the best sort. An early champion of civil rights, Hahn served on LA City Council from 1947 to 1952 and on the County Board of Supervisors for forty consecutive years starting in 1952. It was Hahn who first presented the bill to the legislators who gave their names to it—Assemblyman Larry Townsend and Senator James Wedworth. Hahn was also a close friend of Governor Reagan, the future president, and made a strong case for signing the bill into law. (Hahn was standing over Reagan's left shoulder when the governor signed the legislation; Townsend and Wedworth were witnesses to the Gipper's signature as well.)

I single Hahn out for special praise for a good reason. I sure needed the man to be serving on the Board of Supervisors when I took over the paramedic training program in 1974. It was not only that he was an unwavering supporter of paramedic services; his counsel also kept my patience in place and my temper in check. Gradually, over the four or so years that I ran the training program, we also managed to lower response times in the streets and achieve better health outcomes, including lower death rates for cardiac patients. I spent as much time as possible riding with paramedics to car accidents and other serious health crises. In doing so, I learned by watching them work, only intervening when asked to do so by the crew chief or when I thought I could improve care.

At night, I turned what I learned on the job into a how-to guide on emergency response, often writing at my desk until I nodded off in the wee hours of the morning. My night-owl project, which became the four-volume *Paramedic Training Manuals*, was intended to illustrate specific treatments in the field. The manuals featured my own primitive drawings, simple and illustrative, and language familiar to paramedics. The "textbooks" were used in Los Angeles as a teaching aid in the classroom and a reference manual in the field. I was just happy to write a training document designed specifically for paramedics in the field, who formerly had to learn from texts designed for nurses, physicians, and military medics. (A copy ended up in the Smithsonian Institution's National Museum of American History in 2000, along with several other items from the TV series *Emergency!*, to mark the thirtieth anniversary of the show's premiere.[29])

The LA training program quite literally brought the world to my door. One day, a group of Australian doctors just showed up at my office in LA. The delegation was led by the formidable Bob Wright, whom I considered to be a quintessential Aussie—brash, direct, and charming. Wright and his colleagues proceeded to interrogate me on our paramedic training program. Wright and I were united in some way as citizens of British colonies—though he was a wilder colonial than I could ever pretend to be. We hit it off immediately, and soon enough I was off to Sydney, Australia, to work with his team. The world of emergency medicine, then and now, was a small one, and as word spread about the LA County paramedic training program, I was invited to meet with my colleagues in the Middle East, the United Kingdom, Europe, and Asia as the 1970s progressed. In retrospect, I see that the LA years were formative for me. My peers gave me a much wider perspective on paramedic training and emergency care—none more so than Peter Baskett and Michael Moles, two British nationals who would become lifelong friends. I invited this duo to one of the first, if not *the* first, international conferences on pre-hospital care, which I hosted in Los Angeles in 1977. I knew Baskett was pioneering a promising new analgesic (a mixture of nitrous oxide and oxygen) for pain management in pre-hospital and ambulatory care. Baskett and Moles readily accepted my invitation—the start of decades of collaborations to establish emergency medical services (EMS) as a specialty area of emergency medicine. I would later learn that Moles had a second career as a spy, and that both men were superb speakers. At the time, I was also interested in their role in the Club of Mainz,[30] a group founded in 1976 of emergency-care leaders with a mission to improve pre-hospital and disaster care worldwide.

Here was the other constant in my life In LA: trouble and drama continued to follow me around. For example, I missed taking a ride on another tragic journey—Pacific Southwest Airlines Flight 182 from LA to San Diego on September 25, 1978. The crash killed all 135 people aboard the aircraft and another seven on the ground.[31] I remember the day well. I was characteristically, and in this case luckily, late for the flight, and was not allowed to board the airplane. I was scheduled to deliver a lecture that evening at the University of California campus in San Diego, so I reluctantly rented a car at the airport and headed south. (I hated and still hate freeway driving.) About an hour into the drive, I was half-listening to the radio news when the report of the crash was broadcast. I quickly pulled the car off the freeway, took a deep breath or two, and eventually continued my journey.

Another air tragedy would also get intertwined with my life. After I finished my residency at LAC+USC in 1974, I decided to buy a boat and set up domestic life in a marina. I needed to get away from my twenty-four–hour workdays, and shift work combined with a good salary gave me that option. (I had no time to commute, and less interest in doing so.) My search for a used boat took me to a mansion in a clifftop neighbourhood in Newport Beach. This was quite a place— featuring twin Lamborghinis in the garage, a sunken living room where young women in wispy clothes seemed to act as hosts, and a swimming pool extended atop the cliff, offering an extraordinary view of the blue Pacific. I met the boat's owner, who said he also piloted his own Learjet. This guy was doing okay, I figured, even if he looked like one of those middle-aged guys trying to cling to his youth. (His clothes were just a little too tight and his waist was just a little too thick.) Eventually, I did buy his boat—a Freeport 41, which I moored at Long Beach Marina, just a half-hour drive from the hospital. I named it the *Edith Cavell*, using my mother's first and middle names; Mom herself had been named after British war hero Edith Cavell. (Cavell was a British war nurse who helped about two hundred Allied soldiers escape from Belgium during the First World War. For her efforts, the Germans executed her by firing squad.) The *Edith Cavell* was only nominally my home. I was so busy with my work that I seldom slept there, choosing instead to bed down in on-call rooms at the hospital. I happily let paramedics use the vessel. At times, I fear it became party central. Only a few weeks after I christened the *Edith Cavell*, news broke that a Learjet had crashed near John Wayne Airport, killing four people, including the fellow who'd sold me the boat. Buckets of cocaine were found aboard the airliner, which explains why he could afford his extravagant lifestyle.

I was immediately gripped with fear that the investigation of the accident and the pilot's illegal drug empire would lead to the seizure of the boat I had just bought, so I did what the public relations practitioners say you're supposed to do: I got ahead of the story by calling the Los Angeles County Sheriff's Office, where I served as medical director. I was aboard my houseboat at the time, knew the people at the sheriff's office, and figured a discreet inquiry would follow. About half an hour later, I heard the wail of sirens approaching. A bunch of people jumped out of their cars with a drug-sniffing dog on a leash, ran down the gangplank and promptly handcuffed me to a railing. By then, a crowd of my neighbours had assembled on the wharf while my so-called friends in the sheriff's office proclaimed that they had everything under control. "Don't worry; we got him," they assured the neighbours. No drugs were found on the vessel, by the way, and I ended up paying only a small price for the practical joke my colleagues had played on me. After that very noisy drug raid, my neighbours at the marina gave me a wide berth.

Their cold shoulders, it turns out, were preferable to the warm embrace in which Dr. Jeffrey R. MacDonald tried to encircle me. MacDonald, a former Green Beret captain, was a capable colleague at the County who went on to serve as director of St. Mary Medical Center in Long Beach. When I was preparing to leave LA in 1978 to set up a residency program in emergency medicine at the University of Pittsburgh, Dr. MacDonald was not alone in protesting my departure. He and others—including many firefighters and health professionals who fought my reforms to the paramedic training program—attacked the LA County Board of Supervisors on the mistaken assumption that I was being run out of town. MacDonald himself wrote a blistering letter to Kenneth Hahn, demanding that I retain my positions in La-La

Land. Truth is, I was wrung out after six years in LA, and eager to take on the challenge of setting up a new program in Pittsburgh.

Prior to my departure, MacDonald had sought and obtained permission to return to the east coast to deal with what he called a legal matter. After I moved to Pittsburgh, he asked if he could stop long enough on his coast-to-coast journeys to deliver guest lectures to my residents. Sometime in summer of 1979, he didn't make a scheduled stop on his way back west. The reason quickly became clear enough. On August 29, 1979, MacDonald was convicted of the brutal murders of his wife and two small daughters in 1970 at the family's apartment in Fort Bragg, North Carolina.[32] In that pre-internet era I had no idea that the legal matter that took MacDonald to the east coast was his own murder trial. Others in the LA EMS community, including his employer, St. Mary Medical Center, knew everything about the murder trial. MacDonald—who was handsome, charming, persuasive, and smart—had so convinced his colleagues of this innocence that he actually kept his job until after he was convicted. People even held fundraisers to help pay for his legal defence. I still have one good friend who will insist that his case represents a miscarriage of justice until she is in her grave.

And even after moving to Pittsburgh I would not escape the high-drama episodes that seemed to mark my life.

CHAPTER 7

SCALING NEW HEIGHTS IN PITTSBURGH, 1977–1988

IN 1977, I WAS INVITED TO COME FROM LA TO THE ANNUAL BANQUET OF PENNSYLVANIA AMBU-lance operators, one of those chicken-dinner events that were to become all too common in my life. There, I was approached by Betty Carlson and her husband, Gerald Carlson, a successful Pittsburgh business-man. It was no accident that Betty was in attendance. She worked as a nurse for Don Leon, one of the assistant deans at the medical school at University of Pennsylvania. (He would later become dean.) Betty had clearly been assigned to strike up a conversation with me—in essence to pre-screen me for a possible appointment at the university hospital.

I wasn't so naive that I didn't know what was going on. Quite the contrary: I had diplomatically let it be known that I was looking for new job opportunities. After six years in LA, I had tired of the gnarly medical politics of the great metropolis, with its tangle of relation-ships linking docs, other healthcare professionals, ambulance operators, paramedics, firefighters, politicians, and the Hollywood glitterati. By the mid-1970s I had also made strides by crafting, with my colleagues, a reputable paramedic training program in LA, one recognized by emergency specialists in Australia, New Zealand, and Europe. By the spring of 1977, I was ready to paint on a broader canvas and keen to move closer to home in Nova Scotia. Pittsburgh would take me in the direction I was heading—and the university and its affiliated hospital seemed to provide the kind of academic, research, and clinical settings I was seeking. In short, I was prepared to be wooed and won by the university's medical school.

An approach was made later that year. Don Leon invited me to pay a visit to the campus and to Presbyterian University Hospital. The language of the invitation hardly suggested a firm job offer was about to be tabled, but when I finally travelled to Pittsburgh for my visit in November 1977, I was heartened by the delegation that met me at the airport. Led by the ebullient Betty Carlson, the small group presented me with full winter gear—galoshes, an overcoat, gloves, and a scarf. Pittsburgh couldn't offer me Southern California sunshine, I was being told, but at least I could don survival gear to get through the raw Pennsylvania winters—a remarkable human touch I appreciated. I left Pittsburgh knowing a job was mine for the taking there, though the details would still have to be ironed out. I was pretty sure I wanted to make the move—until I got back to the temperate, blue-sky California winter. Then I began to waver.

There in California, aboard the *Edith Cavell* on a warm and sunny fall day, I took one of the most important phone calls of my life. It was from Dr. Peter Safar, a legend in resuscitation and critical care medicine who would be nominated three times in his life for the Nobel Prize in medicine.[33] Trained as an anesthesiologist, the Austrian-born Safar practised at Johns Hopkins University before setting up a globally recognized resuscitation lab at the University of Pittsburgh. Safar's message to me was simple and direct. In his distinguished Austrian accent, Safar told me that he would back me 100 percent if I took the job in Pittsburgh. He would be my number one cheerleader, come hell or high water. He was also clear about his reasons: Peter wanted to develop his research and clinical program in critical care. He hoped I would take the job to run the then non-existent emergency department and head up EMS. I returned to Pittsburgh to be formally interviewed for the job, and the rest is history.

Emergency medicine, the field in which I trained for three years, would not be recognized as a specialty by US regulators until 1979. In addition, not all my colleagues were keen on my appointment or my field, to say the least. My first dean of medicine at the University of Pittsburgh, Gerhard Werner, made it clear he intended to limit my scope of practice. Why? Well, even in the late 1970s, the medical establishment saw emergency physicians as upstarts and usurpers. Healthcare politics being what they were, people also wanted to hold onto the power they had—not share it with a new service like EMS. In a sense, this was understandable. Before people like Bob Scharf came along, emergency departments were often staffed by docs who couldn't make it in specialties or in family medicine. They were rarely "best in class" as students or "best in practice" as physicians. Werner's successor as dean of medicine, Dr. Gerald Levey, was an academician of the first rank who seemed to disdain the very notion that emergency medicine was a field unto itself. As far as Gerry and his second-in-command, Dr. Mike Karpf, were concerned, I was trespassing on their turf. (Levey's resistance was short-lived. He had a distinguished career and would become the driving force behind the development of the Ronald Reagan UCLA Medical Center.[34] We would later reunite over the occasional dinner and conversation in his UCLA office, before his death in 2021.)

Given the ambivalence among a few of the senior staff doctors toward my appointment at the University of Pittsburgh medical school, it was no wonder that my recruitment had been something of a clandestine affair.

But then came the rescue of Ralph Winner Jr.

Just before noon on a damp, overcast spring morning in Pittsburgh, I took the call. It was May 23, 1978, three weeks after I had started my new jobs as a professor of medicine at the University of Pittsburgh and director of the emergency department at the Presbyterian University Hospital. An ironworker was trapped between two structural girders high above the city. Ralph Winner Jr. had been working on the demolition of the Brady Street Bridge, a century-old span that rose 127 feet above the Monongahela River. Winner, a member of Ironworkers Local Union #3, had twenty-seven years of experience in his trade. On that fateful day, he was teamed up with Don Zeller, a work partner for more than three decades. Both men were using acetylene torches to cut slits in the girders. Explosives were going to be set in the slits and detonated sometime in June. Zeller would later report that his friend had been sitting on a girder, gazing down toward the river through lightly falling rain, when the bridge had suddenly shifted.[35] A bridge span had given way, trapping Winner's legs just below the knee. A fleet of paramedic and firefighter vehicles quickly converged on the scene, clogging the northbound lanes of the adjacent Birmingham Bridge, which had been opened in 1976 to replace the Brady Street structure.

I was in my apartment when I took the call from the shift supervisor in the emergency medical services department, who briefed me on the incident. He said he would pick me up in a few minutes. To get out of my apartment, I stepped through the maze of cardboard boxes littering the floor, still unopened from the move. By the time I got to the front door, the EMS vehicle was already waiting, so I jumped into the passenger seat and we raced toward the Birmingham Bridge, sirens on and lights flashing.

It was clear I would have to get a close look to assess the patient's condition. That meant climbing a hundred-foot ladder in a slight mist. I had conquered an aversion to heights at rescue scenes while working from ladders in LA, but this ascent might well have induced lifelong acrophobia. For the first thirty feet or so, it felt as if I was just walking up a set of steps with railings to hold on both sides. Focussed on the task at hand, I didn't notice that the last two-thirds of the steep climb were more perilous. Soon I found myself grasping for handholds that were no longer there and fell face-first into a plain old ladder. I steadied myself and continued the ascent, trying not to look down. When I inevitably did, I saw a crowd gathering on the Birmingham Bridge, framed by the steely waters of the Monongahela River below. As the *Pittsburgh Press* reported the next day: "When faced with the 100-foot climb up an aerial ladder to reach Winner, Stewart said he didn't look down into the murky waters. 'I kept repeating the Hippocratic Oath and thinking of the man who needed help,' Stewart said."

The paramedics who preceded me to the scene had done everything by the book. They had administered morphine to Winner and taken a blood sample so it could be crossed and matched to get the right blood type for possible transfusions. Paramedics had already told me by radio that there was no evidence Winner was in shock. An IV was started to provide vascular access for giving drugs and fluids. I had ordered O negative blood from the hospital, although it never arrived. (Out-of-hospital blood was rarely considered an option to transfuse patients at that time.) Fortunately, though Winner was in severe pain, his blood pressure and other vital signs were normal, so no transfusions were required.

I called Joe Young, the senior surgical resident then rotating through the emergency department, and instructed him to bring a surgical tray and a Gigli saw to the scene. Useful particularly for amputations, the cutting edge of the Gigli is a flexible, sharpened wire attached to T-shaped handles at both ends. While Winner remained trapped, his fellow ironworkers were using acetylene torches to cut the girder entrapping his legs. Incredibly, he had attempted to do this himself when the accident first happened. One leg had been freed, and we hoped to release the second one, though it was not clear that either limb could be saved.

But then the bridge shifted again, ever so slightly.

I looked down and saw that officials from the state were huddled under a bright red umbrella. Within minutes, the workers were told to put down their torches. Representatives from the Department of Transportation had calculated the risk of cutting the beam that trapped Winner's legs. David Spagnolli, a stress control engineer with the state of Pennsylvania, concluded that the two beams trapping Winner met at a critical stress point.[36] If the beams were separated, the bridge could collapse—quite possibly onto the adjacent Birmingham Bridge. Workers and the rescue team could plunge to their deaths into the river.

At that point, Winner, lucid throughout his agonizing ordeal, understood that the only option was an amputation of his leg at the knee. He consented to the procedure. It was time for Joe Young to spring into action. In medical parlance, the procedure Joe performed on the high girders is called a disarticulation of the knee, but "amputation" has a clearer meaning to lay audiences. I can live with that term, but I resist the common reportorial phrase, "The doctor cut his leg off." That language leads people to imagine a power saw ripping through bone. In fact, no bone is cut during this procedure. We would use the Gigli saw to cut through the ligaments and tissues surrounding the knee joint, avoiding the upper (femur) and lower (tibia) bones of the leg. Young performed the surgery quickly and skillfully. Winner was sedated using morphine and diazepam, the only medications available to our team. The challenge was to balance the need to maintain his breathing while dulling his sensitivity to pain.

Winner was lowered from the girders by crane at 3:20 P.M. and taken to Presbyterian University Hospital, which was quite near the scene. There, Winner's wife, Jean, and his brother Dick kept a vigil outside the Intensive Care Unit alongside his fellow ironworkers, who paid brief visits to their union brother as he recuperated. I was able to drop by to see Winner from time to time as his treatment progressed.

I was more medical supervisor than action hero in the Brady Street Bridge story. The latter designation rightly belongs to Joe Young, the paramedics, and the ironworkers who helped keep Winner alive. As the physician ultimately responsible for the emergency response, however, I became the public face and voice of the bridge rescue story in local and national media, doing three or four interviews a day for the best part of a fortnight. I was approached by the Kiwanis organization, which asked if I would accept its Star of Courage Award. I agreed—on the condition that the entire medical team receive the award; I was only one of eight or so people who treated Winner, and he may not have survived his ordeal had paramedics not taken the proper treatment measures before I arrived on the scene.

The media fame I earned, or endured, from the bridge incident gave me a key to the city, and I was quick to turn it. I had learned in LA that a celebrity profile can open a lot of doors in America, and I leveraged my "fifteen minutes of fame" to highlight the importance of EMS in the Pittsburgh area and beyond.

The context is important here. I had been hired as the director of the emergency department, which sounds grand enough, but in fact I was the sole physician permanently assigned to said emergency department, and I was marching blind into a frontier. I was also appointed head of EMS in Pittsburgh, another job in which I flew solo as one of the few physicians (if not the only one) in Pennsylvania who had been through a residency program in emergency medicine. For my first two years in Pittsburgh, I would be constantly on call to support paramedics in the field, either giving orders directly over radio, or monitoring what orders were being given by residents rotating through the university hospital emergency department. I literally slept with a radio.

After the bridge rescue, I approached hospitals affiliated with the University of Pittsburgh to raise additional money for a new centre for emergency medicine, seeking an average contribution of about $130,000 per year from each. CEOs actually called me to get involved and, in the end, almost everyone I approached signed up. Within six months of my arrival in Pittsburgh, the Center for Emergency Medicine was up and running.[37] Today, the world-renowned centre remains dedicated to improved pre-hospital care and operates a fleet of helicopters and emergency vehicles which transport more than nine thousand patients per year.

Launching the centre was crucial—it literally institutionalized emergency health services in the city. It also enabled our small community of EHS providers and supporters to entrench research and educational programs in emergency care. I also believed, after my years in LA, that I knew what a comprehensive EHS system would look like. My California dream years allowed me to reach out well beyond what my role in emergency medical care could be. The paramedic training program I had launched in LA was successful enough that it took me all over the world. By the time I got to Pittsburgh, I had literally written the book on how it should be done. I knew how organizations and bureaucracies worked and had learned how to deal with them. I knew I might have a role to play in forming the specialty known as emergency medicine and was directing myself toward that end.

At the same time, I found myself with little initial support to get the job done. I also learned, to my chagrin, that the politics of EMS services were as thorny in Pittsburgh as they had been in LA. Even my persuasive recruiter, Peter Safar, was at the centre of a storm—so much so that, while I was confident he had my back, I wondered who had his. In the years before my arrival in Pittsburgh, Peter had been in a battle royal with the powerful mayor, Peter Flaherty, a flamboyant populist from the city's Irish American community, who ran the city with an iron fist. The issue that divided the two Peters was support for Freedom House, an African American institution that served the Black community in a city deeply split along racial lines.[38] Flaherty was determined to withdraw funding for the institution. Safar and his colleagues fought to the end for Freedom House, which was forced to close in 1975. (Safar and Philip Hallen were the visionary leaders who established an ambulance service through Freedom House in 1967.)

Safar trained marginalized underemployed or unemployed people as medical technicians and ambulance operators. His three-hundred–hour course offered a training curriculum that included not only cardiac care but also advanced first aid training, nursing, defensive driving, anatomy, and physiology.[39] This was clearly groundbreaking: the paramedics operating out of Freedom House in the late 1960s may have deployed a wider set of skills than virtually any other first responders on the planet. (The Irish innovators in Dublin and Belfast had designed ambulance systems with a narrower scope of out-of-hospital treatment in mind, focussed on cardiac patients.)

Safar and Hallen clearly understood the link between good health-care outcomes and economic success—and the ambulance service could help deliver both. Other key players who shared this understanding included Dr. Don Benson, the founding medical director of Freedom House, and Dr. Nancy Caroline, who would later become a driving force behind the development of the Freedom House ambulance service.[40] Benson and Caroline, who both studied under Safar, helped build Freedom House's reputation as a pioneer in the delivery of quality care in the streets. (Caroline also wrote the landmark textbook *Emergency Care in the Streets*, which is still in print.)

Safar's background helps explain his passion in the battle with Flaherty and the city. Born in 1924 in Austria, he knew first-hand about racism: he had to conceal his Jewish heritage to evade persecution by the Nazis in the 1930s. He could see that African American people in his adopted city of Pittsburgh were benefitting from and proud of the Freedom House ambulance service. In addition, his own daughter Elizabeth had died of an asthma attack at age eleven, after she was transported to a hospital in an emergency vehicle without being treated en route.[41]

Safar minced no words when the mayor proposed to yank funding from Freedom House. In an open letter, Safar and Benson lambasted

Mayor Flaherty's administration for allowing police to interfere with paramedics as they treated patients in the streets, calling the city's approach to ambulance services a "disgrace."[42] Traditionally, police officers had served as first responders in Pittsburgh—they saw it as part of their job to put patients in a vehicle and drive as quickly as possible to a hospital to deliver their charges into care. In fairness, it should be stated that Flaherty's goal wasn't to return EMS service to the bad old days, but to replace the Freedom House model with a city-operated service. Safar's battle on behalf of Freedom House may have put him on the side of the angels, but it didn't endear him to the university or the hospital he served, both of which depended on good relations with City Hall. Fortunately for me, and for Safar, Flaherty took an appointment as President Jimmy Carter's attorney general in 1977, and his attention was diverted. Yet, I was keenly aware Washington wasn't far from Pittsburgh, and Flaherty still wielded power in the city. I was wary of the aftershocks from the Freedom House battle when I first arrived in the city, as I tried to build on the foundations and personnel remaining from the struggles they had waged.

When I arrived in Pittsburgh I was a little intimidated—at first—by Dr. Thomas Detre, the university's senior vice chancellor for the health sciences.[43] Like Safar, he had been born in central Europe (Hungary) in 1924. To me, he felt like European royalty. He spoke elegant English with a distinct Austro-Hungarian accent. He carried a cigarette holder with a cigarette always in place but never lit. The cigarette holder was rapier-like and intimidating, depending on how vigorously the senior vice chancellor would wave it about. It took me a few meetings with him to realize it was all part of his act—though an impressive one. When I first arrived in Pittsburgh, he invited me to a brief meeting. I was fairly certain no wet-behind-the-ears recent hire at Pitt was usually

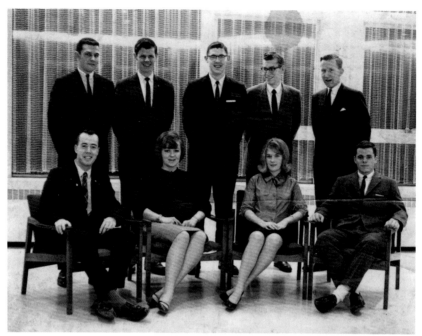

Ron Stewart (front row, far left) ran for president of the Acadia students' union in 1964–65. Protests against the Vietnam War were just starting to heat up in the US, and Stewart positioned his campaign as a protest against student apathy. The "yes" vote was 97 percent in favour. (AUTHOR COLLECTION)

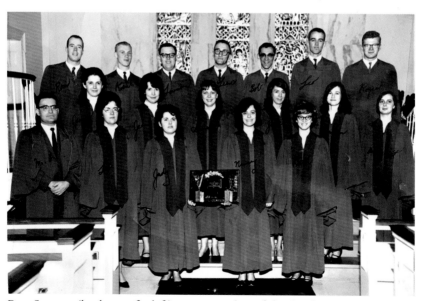

Ron Stewart (back row, far left) was a member of the Acadia University choir, which won a national competition in 1965. (AUTHOR COLLECTION)

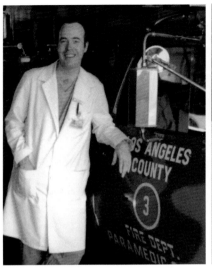
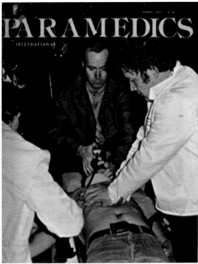

LEFT: Ron Stewart with an LA Paramedic Squad vehicle; a similar vehicle appeared on the TV show *Emergency!* (AUTHOR COLLECTION)

RIGHT: One evening in 1976 as Ron Stewart travelled back to LA from a meeting in the San Fernando Valley he stopped at the scene of a car crash, intervening at the request of the paramedics on site. This image made the cover of *Paramedics International* magazine. (RICK MCCLURE)

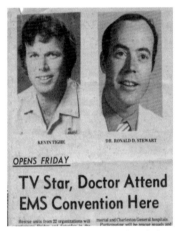
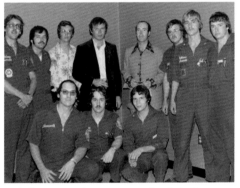

LEFT: Ron Stewart, medical director of paramedic training for LA County, and Kevin Tighe, star of *Emergency!*, were special guests at the West Virginia EMS convention in 1976. (AUTHOR COLLECTION)

RIGHT: Actor Kevin Tighe (brown jacket), who played paramedic/firefighter Roy DeSoto on *Emergency!*, often travelled with Ron Stewart (shown here in what he calls the "unfortunate blue leisure suit") to promote the show and the profession of paramedicine. This photo was taken at the West Virginia Paramedics Championship in 1976. (AUTHOR COLLECTION)

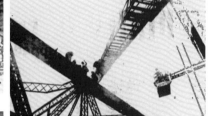
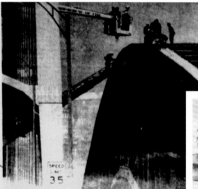

On May 23, 1978, ironworker Ralph Winner Jr. was working on the demolition of the Brady Street Bridge in Pittsburgh when the structure shifted and trapped his legs between two girders. These images show Ralph Winner being rescued by a medical team led by Ron Stewart—working a hundred feet in the air. *(PITTSBURGH PRESS, FREE-LANCE STAR)*

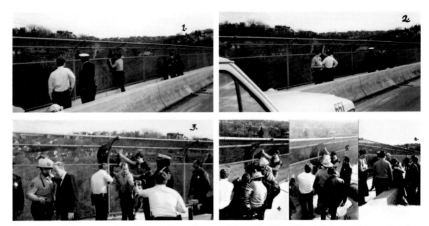

Pittsburgh's many bridges often figured in EMS calls. This call involved a young hospital food services worker intent on jumping to the freeway below. He asked for Ron Stewart specifically because Stewart was one of the few people who greeted him in the cafeteria line. In the third frame, he is seen clinging to side of the fence. As the last frame shows, he was eventually persuaded to climb back to safety. Stewart is standing directly behind the two people who are embracing. (AUTHOR COLLECTION)

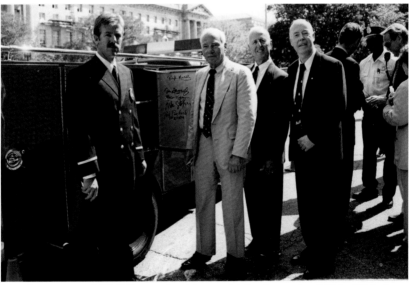

The "pioneers of EMS" stand with a vehicle from the 1970s TV show *Emergency!* that was donated to the Smithsonian in 2000 by "Project 51," an organization established to celebrate the thirtieth anniversary of paramedic training program in the US. In the light suit, Dr. Michael Criley; Drs. Eugene Nagel and Ronald Stewart stand to the right. (AUTHOR COLLECTION)

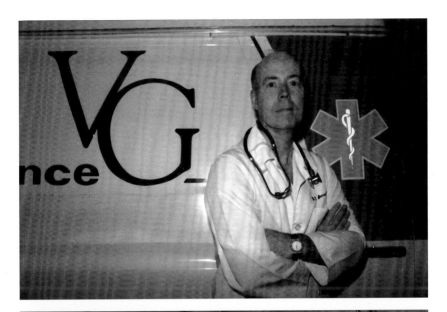

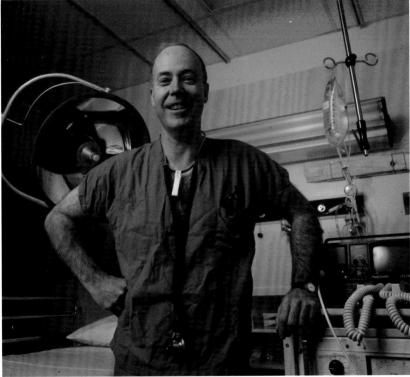

Nova Scotia called in 1989 when the head of anesthesiology at Dalhousie University offered Ron Stewart a job in emergency medicine in Halifax.
(MICHAEL CREAGAN)

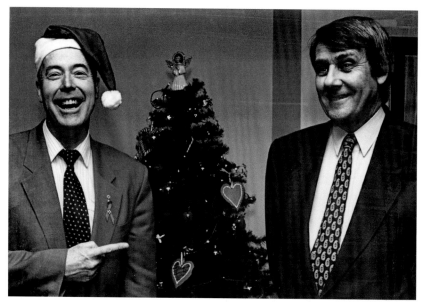

Minister of Health Ron Stewart (left) joking with Deputy Minister Armand Pinard as they pose for the newsletter Christmas photo, 1995. (AUTHOR COLLECTION)

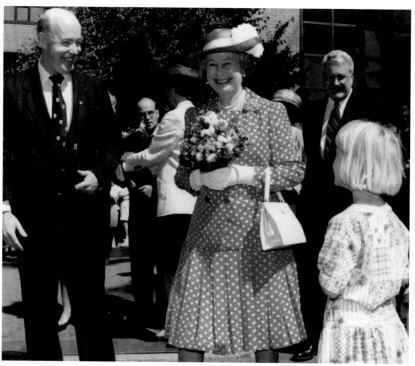

In August 1994, Queen Elizabeth and Prince Philip visited Halifax, where the queen opened the new Queen Elizabeth II Health Sciences Centre. Health Minister Ron Stewart is shown at left; Premier John Savage is in the background, right. (AUTHOR COLLECTION)

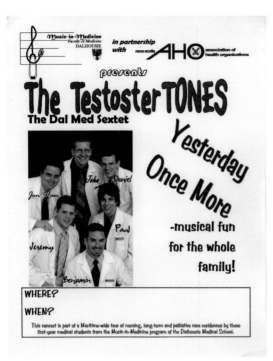

Music-in-Medicine
Faculty of Medicine
DALHOUSIE

in partnership with
nova scotia AHO association of health organizations

presents

The TestosterTONES
The Dal Med Sextet

John   Daniel
Jon-athan
Jeremy   Paul
Benjamin

Yesterday Once More

-musical fun for the whole family!

WHERE?

WHEN?

This concert is part of a Maritime-wide tour of nursing, long-term and palliative care residences by these first-year medical students from the Music-in-Medicine program of the Dalhousie Medical School.

As director of the Music in Medicine program at Dalhousie University in the early 2000s, Ron Stewart put together a popular men's singing group known as the Testostertones. Stewart's predecessor, Thomas John (Jock) Murray, held the core belief that physicians need to understand human beings to be good at their jobs, and music was a key part of that. (AUTHOR COLLECTION)

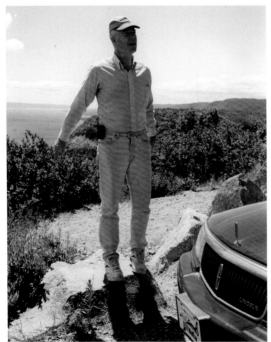

Ron Stewart takes in the view from Cape Smokey during a roadside stop in Cape Breton, July 2000. (AUTHOR COLLECTION)

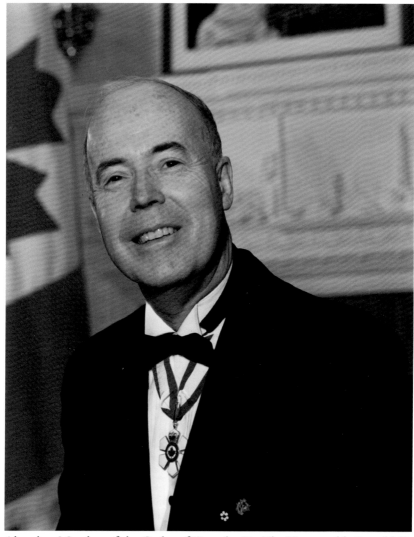

Already a Member of the Order of Canada, Dr. The Honourable Ronald D. Stewart, CC, ONS, ECNS, MD, was elevated to Companion of the Order of Canada on November 14, 2023, for his groundbreaking contributions to the field of emergency medicine and for his sustained leadership in the public health sector. (GEORGE GEORGAKAKOS)

interviewed by the vice chancellor. I suspected it meant that Detre was sizing me up as to whether I could calm the stormy waters between the city, the mayor, and Dr. Safar, rather than how slick I was at placing an endotracheal tube or slipping in an IV line.

He told me we would meet annually for a sandwich and a drink afterward—either water or whiskey. Whiskey meant I had his approval to serve for another year. The other libation meant I was water under the bridge. At the end of that first meeting, he poured each of us a whiskey and said, "You're good for the first year anyway." Despite his Old World charm, Detre was determined to keep the very best people at the university, and he would fire those who didn't meet his standards. (We were all appointed "at will"—to use the British parliamentary phrase that describes cabinet appointments—and could be fired at will without recourse.) He was an extraordinary leader and positioned the university as one of the nation's top ten recipients of federal healthcare funding. Every year of my tenure in Pittsburgh, he poured me a shot of whiskey at the end of our annual meeting. He was consistently a strong supporter of my work. Without Tom Detre's backing, I never would have accomplished anything at the university. (When I finally told him I was quitting my position to return to Canada, I think he even got a little emotional— though he was hardly the sort of man to cry into his whiskey.)

Only once during my decade in Pittsburgh did Detre summon me to an impromptu meeting. On the way to the office, I thought to myself, "This can't be good news." And sure enough, it wasn't. It turned out that one of my senior colleagues was having an affair with a woman in our department. I have always been naive about this sort of thing and was the last person to know what was going on. I left Detre's office with instructions straight out of a spy novel. I was to talk to my colleague and call Detre back to utter one word: Yes. That would mean that the problem was dealt with. I went straight to the offender's office; he immediately confessed that the rumour was true and said he would sort it all out. Relieved, I made the call to Detre. My colleague soon departed to take a position at a medical school out of state. I mention this affair to confess a weakness and admit the area of my work in which I was least skilled; I was ready for almost everything as a leader in emergency medicine—except the thorny human relations. Frankly, I retained a naïveté about workplace politics, workplace relationships, and workplace rivalries that didn't serve anyone well. In a sense, my Calvinist religious upbringing—or indoctrination—had worked all too well. I tended to think the best of everyone and often suffered for doing so.

All that said, this colleague's departure was a loss for me. Happily, I was able to build a base of support within and beyond the confines of the hospital. To accomplish the latter, I put on a road show, accepting invitations to speak before business, community, educational, and healthcare organizations in Pittsburgh and the surrounding areas of eastern Ohio and western Pennsylvania. One evening while driving to an event, something unusual happened: I suddenly started to shake and sweat. My heart was racing and my breathing was laboured. I pulled over and stopped at the side of the road in the pouring rain. After I recovered somewhat, I realized that my windshield wipers had triggered a traumatic memory of my accident north of Smokey Mountain, Cape Breton Island. The wipers would have been swishing back and forth on that fateful spring night in 1971 when I drove off the highway and suffered a serious brain injury. Now, years later, I was clearly experiencing an episode of post-traumatic stress disorder (PTSD) as I drove toward my engagement. Luckily, nothing like that has happened since. I did manage to carry out my speaking commitment.

It seemed everyone in Pennsylvania wanted to hear about the bridge rescue, and I had told the story often enough that I could almost deliver the performance on automatic pilot. What I wanted to talk about was effective EMS—which depended on quick response times, paramedics trained in resuscitation, quality pre-hospital care overall, and taking the patients to the right hospitals for treatment.

In Pennsylvania, as in most US states, people immediately understood the continuum-of-care argument because there was a story to go with it. When Governor David L. Lawrence died in 1966, more than a fortnight after collapsing from a heart attack at a political rally, Pittsburgh ambulances were staffed by police officers who drove patients to hospital. Care started at the hospital door—not soon enough for Lawrence and many other patients.[44] This had started to change in 1967, the year after Lawrence's death, when the Freedom House ambulance service was established in Pittsburgh.

By the time I arrived in Pittsburgh, there was a clamour to extend city-quality EMS services to people in outlying areas. As a result, my road show—advocating better emergency response services—was well received. It helped that I received great overall support from Mayor Richard Caliguiri, who had succeeded Peter Flaherty at City Hall. Hospital administrators who had supported the Center for Emergency Medicine were also onboard—none more helpfully than Dan Stickler, then the CEO of Presbyterian University Hospital. (Stickler was a close ally who became a close friend. He was intrigued by my descriptions of my Cape Breton home—which didn't endear me to everyone—and more than once travelled to the island to visit my parents.)

All this was happening in the late 1970s and early 1980s, the pioneering era of emergency medical response flights. Helicopters were all the rage, and as hospitals competed to attract patients, every hospital wanted its own chopper and helipad as part of the product offering. The scope of my job became much broader than I had expected. It was presumed my excursions beyond the city would attract patients to the university hospitals, and helicopter transport was part of my sales pitch in smaller communities surrounding Pittsburgh.

Competition is an integral part of the US healthcare system: attract more patients, provide more care, and you generate more revenue. It's a simple formula. But I'm an MD, not an MBA, and my motive was not beating the pants off Allegheny General Hospital, which had introduced its LifeFlight helicopter earlier in the 1970s. I knew I needed to play a long game here, with a goal not of winning a political war but of providing better integrated care to patients—from the scene of an accident, through the transport stage, into the emergency department, and on to the hospital wards. We did introduce a helicopter service under what we called the Specialized Treatment and Transport (STAT) program.

As a name, STAT isn't nearly as market friendly as LifeFlight, but our service did enjoy what advertising executives call a market differentiator. LifeFlight, as the name implies, was clearly about moving people by air. Helicopter delivery of patients was sexy in the early days, but it could kill them if continuum of care wasn't provided, or if patients were delivered to hospitals that (for instance) had no blood for transfusions. STAT was about transporting patients by the most appropriate means possible, which inevitably meant surface transportation on foggy or windy or stormy days. The people of Pittsburgh, after all, are no strangers to inclement weather. Our focus on moving patients on days when helicopters couldn't fly was a clear benefit to patients. So was our decision to transport patients to the nearest hospitals that could competently and professionally treat people—regardless of whether they were Pitt-affiliated institutions. Once again, the emphasis was on *integrated* care.

My strategy required patience; it would take time to execute and time to succeed. It would also require well-trained healthcare professionals. We needed to get more people trained in paramedic care, and in a profession in which it is often difficult to clearly define the indices of success, I take some satisfaction in reporting that several state colleges started offering courses in emergency medicine during my decade in Pittsburgh. Allegheny College was an early adopter, setting up emergency medical technician programs at the junior college level. Fire departments began to take note of the trend and sponsored their own upgrade programs for first responders. It was a clear example of success breeding success.

Just as importantly, many of the paramedics trained during my years in Pittsburgh and LA became educators and mentors themselves. At least four earned PhDs and became leaders and educators in their field. One of them, Gregg Margolis, would later serve as the director of health policy fellowships at the National Academy of Medicine. We also used our day-to-day delivery of pre-hospital care as a sort of research experiment. This wasn't in-laboratory or control-group scientific research, but the kind based in real experience. We looked at what worked best in responding to a cardiac incident or in transporting patients with apparent spinal injuries or in dealing with the anxieties of patients and loved ones. We talked about these issues every day, analyzing what worked and what didn't. In paramedic medicine, then and now, the streets were a living laboratory.

Our success in putting the STAT principles into practice depended crucially on support from other doctors. Initially, not everyone in the University of Pittsburgh system wanted to see us succeed. Happily, Henry (Hank) Bahnson and Tom Starzl understood what continuous, integrated care meant and wanted to be a part of it.[45] [46] Bahnson, the head of surgery when I was in Pittsburgh, was what my parents would have called "a steady pair of hands." Soft-spoken, patient, and resolute, Bahnson diplomatically put my case before hospital administrators and university executives. I could not have had a better ally. Starzl was also a superstar—a pioneering transplant surgeon, who unlike Bahnson liked seeing his meteor flame across the nocturnal firmament. Flamboyant and outspoken, he was a good man to have on your side. If you were a hospital bean-counter or executive, it was hard to argue with a guy who attracted wealthy patients from all over the world to your hospital for care. Despite their contrasting personalities, Bahnson and Starzl were close friends who shared one view: the patients who finally came under their watch (and their scalpels) should arrive at the hospital in the best possible condition. That was where their goals and mine clearly aligned, and it explained their dogged support of STAT.

To be honest, some of that success was more illusory than real. Andrew Schneider, a reporter with the *Pittsburgh Press* who would win two Pulitzer Prizes before he died in 2017, saw through the illusion all too clearly.[47] He was a formidable public interest reporter, and I was afraid of him. Andy asked all the right questions, and candid answers could have put my job and my career in jeopardy. Emergency medicine was getting a lot of public attention during my years in Pittsburgh, but who were these heroes staffing the emergency department at University-Presbyterian, anyway? Were they well trained? And what were the standards of care? Honest answers to these questions were troubling. On staffing: "No heroes here, only a rotating group of residents thrown into the fray, and me as the only trained emergency doc in the place." On training: "It was on-the-job-training—learn as you go." On standards: "The best standards we could meet, given the experience level of residents."

Schneider wanted to expose all this, and he was anything but shy about using me as a source. I could have stonewalled him, but I didn't see much sense in that strategy. He was a notoriously persistent reporter, not about to go away because I had taken a vow of silence. (He had put in so many unscheduled appearances at Allegheny General Hospital in Pittsburgh that staff finally gave him a lab coat along with a Dr. Schneider name tag.[48]) Andy also had the best of motives—he wasn't a "gotcha" journalist but a reporter acting in the public interest. Shine a little light on EMS in Pittsburgh, he thought, and the health administrators might just improve standards of training and care. In short, we held the same views and wanted to achieve the same ends.

I became his unnamed source; he became a public advocate for better EHS. I also struck a tacit agreement with my dean at the time, Don Leon, that this arrangement was acceptable. Better to bring Andy Schneider into the tent as much as we could than to have him firing missiles at us from outside. Our relationship became oddly symbiotic. I used to tell him. "I hate you, Andy, because you scare me, and love you because you're moving things forward." Schneider also had a knack for telling a story in a way that kept me out of trouble while advancing important issues like professional standards of care. He applied pressure constantly and turned up the heat slowly.

The public focus on emergency healthcare, both positive and critical, did help me recruit new talent to the emergency medical team in Pittsburgh. Dr. Paul Paris followed me from LA to Pittsburgh in 1980 after he had just completed a fellowship in emergency medicine at Cedars-Sinai Medical Center in Los Angeles. His reputation suggested he was a first-rate clinician, which would prove to be the case through his long and storied career. At that time, however, Paul's resumé didn't reflect great depth on the research side—his most recent publication related to fracture of the penis. Our interview panel was chaired by Dr. Joanne Marie Andiorio (who was also a Catholic nun) and included the erudite William Robinson, a surgeon of some renown and an expert on Scotch whiskies to boot. Andiorio and Robinson were sitting side by side when Robinson fired a loaded question at Paris: "Is fracture of the penis your only research interest, Dr. Paris?" Paris deadpanned a one-word response: "Yes." Andiorio, whom I knew well, would have chuckled to herself at the witticism. Yes, she was a Catholic nun, but as the CEO of Mercy Hospital, she was also a woman wise to the world.

We hired Paris, and this proved to be a great decision. Paul was driven to provide quality care and was the leader in implementing many of the systemic reforms to the EMS system in the late 1970s and early 1980s, including the introduction of a residency program in emergency medicine at the University of Pittsburgh. In 1988, the year

I returned to Canada, Paul took on much of the work I had started. As I write this, early in 2023, he is still serving as a professor emeritus there. When we took Paris on in 1980, though, all I knew was that we needed him.

Our second recruit was also an important addition to the department. Mike Heller also crossed the country from California to join our team in 1984. Heller would say anything to anyone, and his brash outspokenness was, to me at least, a virtue. Mike was more than willing to be interviewed by Schneider, was tough enough and valuable enough to withstand any blowback from hospital administrators and was sometimes too open with media. Once, after watching police botch a rescue effort on one of the city's rivers, he blew a gasket in front of reporters. Dr. Levey, my chief of service, once told me to fire Heller for talking openly to reporters—and expressing his opinions to all regardless of where they fit in the medical hierarchy. I replied, for the only time in my career, that if Heller had to go, I was going with him. The chief backed down. I had good reasons to keep Heller around. Like Paris, he was a first-class clinician who would become a pioneer in the use of hand-held ultrasound devices in emergency care. (As I write this, Heller is still practising at Mount Sinai Hospital in New York.)

In Pittsburgh, we made steady progress in the delivery of quality emergency care, but not without dramatic setbacks. No incident hit us harder or revealed more serious gaps in emergency care than the death of a beloved colleague. Walter (Wally) Grubbs, a twenty-six-year-old paramedic, died from his injuries in a car accident two miles outside the Pittsburgh city limits, just after his small vehicle collided with a station wagon that had crossed the centre line on August 28, 1986. Grubbs was a skilled paramedic and leader, a man who had advocated for better emergency services laws before state legislative committees, and a professional so clear-headed in a crisis that he was advising the emergency crew that showed up to help him. Sadly, the suburban medics who came to his rescue badly needed that advice; overall, the emergency system's response was a tragedy of errors. An initial call for a helicopter was reportedly not received, and Grubbs was taken to a hospital (Homestead Emergency and Family Medicine Center) that did not have blood supplies to transfuse him.

Afterward, my comments to the media were so harsh that I'm pretty sure they would have gotten me fired earlier in my tenure at Pittsburgh. I told the *Pittsburgh Press* I found it "painfully hard to accept that a facility that accepts trauma patients does not have blood available at all times."[49] I noted that Wally's death underlined the importance of the battle he fought for improved medical services.

"It was exactly what Wally…was frightened of—that no one was really examining or controlling the EMS system to ensure that it worked, that lives that could be saved weren't being lost."

As I relive the Pittsburgh years in my mind, I realize my closest friendships were with colleagues like Wally—that is, with my work colleagues. People speak of the value of work–life balance, but my life was made all the richer by the integration of both. I even shared my home, which I rarely visited myself, with paramedics, nurses, residents, and others who might have wanted a place to sleep between overtime shifts. I had purchased a home in the tony neighbourhood of Squirrel Hill, where the political elite tended to cluster. As with my houseboat in LA, this home was used more often by my colleagues than by me. I often slept in a call room at the hospital, one of the small cell-like bedrooms where on-call residents grabbed a little shut-eye while putting in their shifts. I had bought the residence only because my secretary said it would be useful to do so financially. (Mortgage interest is deductible against income tax in the US, a tax advantage Canadians do not enjoy.) One day, after a long series of overtime calls in the streets, I returned home to find an elderly woman I had never seen before furiously sweeping the floor in the kitchen.

"Who are you?" she asked.

"I own the place," I replied.

She never paused her sweeping.

I then wandered into the living room where a man who seemed to be lying on the couch jumped up when I entered and started sweeping the floor himself.

I more or less ignored them, thinking some of my guests had hired the pair to clean house. I was mistaken, though, and the mystery was only cleared up a few days later when I took a call from the Pittsburgh police. "Dr. Stewart, there are two people living in your house who have escaped from Mayview." Mayview was the state hospital for psychiatric patients. I was asked if I wanted to press charges. I said no, I just wanted them to take the poor souls back to the hospital, where I hoped they would get the care they needed. (They weren't going to get it at my place.) Later, police asked me to sign an affidavit saying the two had been guests in my home. The signature, I was told, would keep the patients off the docket—that is, police would not be compelled to lay charges.

It turned out my home attracted the interest of not only the police but also the mayor. In the lead-up to his re-election in 1981, I took a direct call from Richard Caliguiri, who was my neighbour in Squirrel Hill. Apparently, a group of our fellow neighbours was threatening to picket his house and then proceed to mine. The cause? The appearance of my property, where the uncut lawn resembled something between a field of hay and an alpine meadow. This was one complaint I had to take seriously. Caliguiri was not only a staunch supporter; in my role as director of the city's medical services department, he was also my boss. Eventually, a crew was called in to tame my front-yard wilderness—a mission accomplished only after they had fired up a machine that looked more like a combine harvester than a lawn mower. The neighbours were appeased, and the mayor won re-election handily.

A year later, our department scored a political victory of its own by establishing the university's first residency program in emergency medicine. Paul Paris was the driving force behind this accomplishment. I played a supporting role, but a minor one. In those days, emergency medicine was still an emerging field—even a risky one for residents. Career paths were not clear. Futures were not assured. Pioneers attract some incredible innovators, though, and the six residents we recruited in the program's first year were driven by a passion that made them all leaders in the field. (All of them were still practicing forty years later as I wrote this account).

Two of them, Ronald Roth and Timothy (Leo) Vollmer were also involved in one of the most memorable emergency calls of my decade in Pittsburgh. It came from a school for children with disabilities during the Christmas season of 1983. When the duo showed up at the school, a great wall of sound—wailing and crying—was emitting from one of the classrooms. They entered the class to find Santa Claus—black boots, red suit, white beard, and all—lying on the floor, looking very dead. They immediately commenced CPR, and soon reached a decision to move Santa to the ambulance. (The commotion was understandably upsetting the children.) Inside the ambulance, Bob Zwier, a husky paramedic, pumped Santa's chest to the beat of "Here Comes Santa Claus." This was clearly an ethical breach, and I can only explain Bob's actions in retrospect by keeping in mind that stress and black humour often play supporting roles in serious medical dramas. Back at the hospital, after the patient had been declared dead, Vollmer told Roth that his career was finished: "After all, you've killed Santa Claus." Roth, a devout Jew, didn't miss a beat in responding, "Right—you're going to blame us for that, too."

The story then took a turn from the absurd to the sublime. Zwier was nowhere to be found. Where had he gone? To buy a Santa suit. The next day, he donned it and drove back to the school to finish giving the kids their presents. He would play that role for a dozen more years. As the physician overseeing this trio, I may have had some obligation to investigate any possible ethical breaches and reprimand appropriately.

I chose what I hoped was the better part of wisdom—a gentle reminder to all concerned that, although something had clearly gone amiss when the trio killed Santa, something had gone terribly right as well. As Vollmer later remarked, Zwier's decision to play Santa represents "the pinnacle of what we're supposed to be."

By the mid-1980s, the time had come for me to head north. In 1980, emergency medicine had finally been recognized as a specialty in Canada, so a market was opening up for people with my background and experience.

In 1987, I was approached directly by officials from Sunnybrook Hospital in Toronto, where the University of Toronto's trauma unit— the biggest and best in the country—was located. A recruiting team flew down from Toronto, wined and dined me and offered me a job. I knew there was a good team in place in emergency services in Pittsburgh. Heller and Paris were both first-rate clinicians, capable leaders, and strong advocates for EHS. Our residents were top drawer. I knew I would be leaving the university, the hospital, and the Center for Emergency Medicine in good hands when I agreed to take a workaday job as a clinician at Sunnybrook.

I was excited to be planning my long-awaited journey toward my home in Canada. I was ready to focus not on building a team but on working on one; not on training new paramedics but on learning from experienced ones; not on navigating the difficult politics of healthcare institutions but on daily clinical practice. I also anticipated that Toronto would be a way station for me, a place to take a deep breath in Canada's largest city before taking a deep dive into the healthcare system in my native province of Nova Scotia—where reform was badly needed.

CHAPTER 8

THE STRANGEST PLACES, 1987-1993

TOWARD THE END OF MY TIME IN TORONTO I WAS CONTACTED BY A COLLEAGUE IN ENGLAND who asked if I might consider coming over to examine the performance of the Sheffield hospital's emergency department in the way they had handled a major incident. The timing was ideal for me and several of the physicians involved were colleagues I had met through my ongoing work with the World Association for Disaster and Emergency Medicine. I signed up and was soon on my way to England and whatever awaited me.

The incident was what became known as the Hillsborough Disaster.

On April 15, 1989, ninety-four people died in a crush of football fans at the Hillsborough Stadium in Sheffield, England. (An additional three people would die later from their injuries.) Football hooliganism had escalated throughout the 1980s in the United Kingdom, and the Hillsborough tragedy was initially seen as another example of fan violence run amok. Four years earlier, in 1985, English clubs had been banned from travelling to Champions League and UEFA Cup (now UEFA Europa) matches on the continent after thirty-nine people died in a riot at Brussels's Heysel Stadium. The deaths occurred after drunken fans of Liverpool FC charged fans from the rival Italian team

Juventus, just before match time on May 29, 1985.[50] A wall collapsed in the fracas. In the wake of the Heysel stadium deaths, Prime Minister Margaret Thatcher and her cabinet supported the ban on British teams travelling to Europe. Thatcher even set up what was described as a war cabinet to deal with football violence inside England.[51]

Given that backstory, it's not surprising that extraordinary steps were taken to keep the Hillsborough match, which also featured the Liverpool side, free of violence. Hillsborough itself was chosen as a neutral venue for the club's FA Cup semi-final match against Nottingham Forest.[52] Extensive efforts were taken to keep rival fans apart. (For instance, supporters of each team were directed to separate entrances at opposite ends of the field.)

Unfortunately, thousands of fans were trapped in "pens" inside the stadium as the match was about to start. Standing-room-only areas were already filled to capacity. When the game got under way, the roar of fans watching the match excited those pushing themselves forward in an attempt to take in every minute of the game. Hundreds of people were being injured or killed in the crush of bodies in the pens, as well as in the densely packed crowds that surged toward the narrow passageway leading to the standing-room-only areas. After six minutes, play was halted when referees and other officials realized what was happening just off the field.

In the immediate aftermath of the tragedy at Sheffield, police officials assigned fault to rampaging fans. Follow-up statements by police and other officials embedded the "drunken hooligan" myth in public consciousness.

And myth it was.

What really caused the deaths?

The Hillsborough deaths were actually caused by poor crowd control, a flawed police response, inadequate preparations for emergency care, and the poor performance of the ambulance service—all compounded by inept communications during the rescue effort. This only became clear in the public mind twenty-three years later. In 2012, an independent panel reported that the tragedy of errors that had occurred in Sheffield was compounded by a police coverup and a misleading coroner's report.[53] The 2012 report found no evidence that either alcohol or unruly fans played a part in the disaster. The panel also concluded that a better rescue effort could have saved at least forty-one lives. In 2016, the jury from a British inquest into the disaster found that ninety-six victims had been "unlawfully killed" at Hillsborough. In 2017, criminal charges were filed against six people—none of them against unruly fans. An additional unlawful death charge was added after attendee Andrew Devine died in 2021 after living for thirty-two years with neurological trauma.

In reviewing the Hillsborough tragedy, I was struck by how many young people were fatally injured. Only seven people older than forty died in the crush, compared to thirty-six kids under twenty. The youngest victim was Jon-Paul Gilhooley, a ten-year-old who had travelled to the stadium with two of his uncles, both of whom survived.[54] Jacqueline Gilhooley would later describe her son as a creative boy who once did his best to paint a bedroom wall with her fingernail varnish. Young Jon-Paul loved football and swimming and watching sports. Gilhooley's tribute to her son served as a reminder to everyone involved in emergency response, and especially in mass-casualty events, that the victims are human, that each human life is precious, and that each patient deserves the best care we can provide. In the chaos of crisis environments involving dozens of people or more, this can be too easily forgotten.

My report and its conclusions can be stated simply—in cases of compression asphyxia, victims tend to either die within minutes or recover quickly. Compression asphyxia defines a condition in which the mechanics of breathing—breathing air/oxygen in and breathing carbon dioxide out—are impossible. The brain quickly becomes depleted of oxygen, and carbon dioxide builds up so that brain activity ceases. Keys to avoiding deaths by compression asphyxia include proper preventive crowd control and correcting conditions that might obstruct breathing. Otherwise, the only real "cure" for this is to relieve the obstructing mechanism to allow breathing. Occasionally, if rescue is rapid and the chest wall is freed from obstruction, recovery can be quick and complete. Occasionally the presence of brain swelling as well as brain damage due to lack of oxygen may be less severe and the patient survives. But then, sadly, survivors may suffer from various levels of brain failure (usually prolonged coma or severe intellectual and physical disabilities). Hospital care at Sheffield, though not particularly challenging, was professional and satisfactory.

Still, I was fully absorbed in my work at Sheffield. It gave me an opportunity, for the first time in decades, to dig into dusty archives and do some historical research. (My inner nerd is captivated by browsing library stacks. I loved the hours I spent throughout my career combing through newspaper archives and medical journals to keep up with my field and conduct my own research, and more recently to recount these experiences.)

There was also an odd serendipity in my assignment in the United Kingdom. It allowed me to take a deep breath after years on the front lines of emergency healthcare as a clinician, educator, and administrator. Sheffield gave me time to ponder my past career and future prospects. I realized then that I could do more to promote improved public health through better and broader emergency care by painting on bigger canvasses (as it were). My prior experience bore this out. I did more to improve emergency healthcare delivery by training hundreds of paramedics in LA than I could have by treating patients one at a time in an emergency department or a clinic. In Pittsburgh, the unlikely bridge story gave me an opportunity to preach my medical gospel about providing better emergency care to a receptive congregation, and my notoriety, as much as I hated to admit it, gave me a receptive audience. I claim only a small measure of credit for the educational and academic infrastructure that was built up in the Pittsburgh area, partially as a result of that outreach effort.

One of the lessons from the Hillsborough Stadium disaster was that architectural design mattered. Build a safer stadium that allows masses of people to reach their seats and depart the venue in an orderly fashion, and you save lives. This notion was hardly new in 1989. More than a century earlier, on June 16, 1883, in Sunderland, England, 183 children had been killed in the Victoria Hall tragedy as they rushed for free toys promised in the wake of a kids' magic show.[55] The victims were trapped and crushed in a pileup behind a single door that opened inward at the bottom of an enclosed stairwell. In the aftermath of the tragedy, an English architect, Robert Alexander Briggs, designed a fastening bolt for theatre doors—the push-bar or panic bolt—which opens the doors from the inside with a forceful shove of a hand or the weight of a body. Some version of Briggs's push bar is now in place, often as a matter of public safety regulations, in tens of thousands of buildings around the world. Briggs, an innovator, architect, and inventor, did more to save lives than any emergency department clinician in the history of the planet.

My experience in England added a chapter to the story I was writing in my head as I began to shape my own philosophy of care or approach to medical practice. If I had to give this unwritten masterpiece a title, it might be *Healthcare is Everybody's Business*. Emergency medical response isn't only about teaching a wide range of people to perform CPR or placing defibrillators in gyms and hockey rinks. It's also about building design, diet, publicly funded healthcare for all, and the notion that it's not only the doctor but also the patient who should respect the old nostrum "heal thyself."

When I had returned to Canada from the US, several years before the Hillsborough event, I had been looking to retreat to clinical practice for a time at Sunnybrook—to get off a treadmill that seemed to move faster and faster during my LA and Pittsburgh years. It sounds shopworn to say this, but my inner Calvinist welcomed the opportunity to provide simple "service" at Sunnybrook. Back home in the "true north, strong and free," I was ready to quietly go back to my origins as a hard-working emergency department physician, providing direct care to patients as part of a team of healthcare professionals. Working with colleagues, learning from some, teaching others, helping patients—that felt like going home to me.

After fifteen tumultuous years in the US, I strove to keep my life simple. A couple of hospital cafeteria meals a day were all the fuel I needed, and I decided to avoid the mistake I'd made in both LA and Pittsburgh, where I had purchased houses in which I rarely lived. In Toronto, my fixed address was the hospital itself, where I was given a small suite in which I could lay my head down on a pillow and catch some rest. I had basically been living in some version of a monk's cell since I'd left home to attend Acadia University in 1960, and the truth was (and is) that I enjoy a simple—what some might consider spartan—lifestyle. I did make some good friends at Sunnybrook, none more memorable than Dafydd (Dave) Rhys Williams, the chief resident who was bright and articulate and wouldn't stop talking about his real goal in life—travelling to outer space.[56] I tried to keep him grounded: "Forget about space, Dave—keep seeing the crowd of patients waiting right here on earth." A decade later, in 1998, I received an invitation to a reception at the Kennedy Space Center in Florida to celebrate a flight of the space shuttle *Columbia*. Dave would be aboard, the first of his two missions in space. Written on my invitation was a simple note in his scrawl: "I told you so."

I had good reasons for not putting down deep roots at Sunnybrook. Toronto was in Canada, all right, but it was only halfway home to Nova Scotia. Prodigal son or not, I had been planning to return to my home soil since the day I'd left the province in 1973 after making a pact with Bob Scharf, and the sooner I could complete the round trip, the better. I had loved living in the US, but despite being surrounded by the warmth of close friends and great colleagues, America was not home.

I was in Toronto less than a year when I was asked to apply for the senior job running the trauma unit and the air ambulance service at Sunnybrook. Colleagues told me a refusal to apply for the job would not be career-enhancing, given the politics of the place. I was selected to do the job, and again became a leader in emergency medicine—this time a restless one. I found myself driving home to Cape Breton again and again—a twenty-one hour endurance test.

On one of those trips, at twilight on a cool autumn evening, I came across an accident near Kingston, about two hours east of Toronto on Highway 401. A man driving a pickup truck in the westbound lane lost control of his vehicle before it hit the median. I was headed east, and I vividly recall the front lights of the pickup shining into the sky briefly before the car flipped and the rear lights illuminated the heavens. The car rolled over repeatedly, creating a light show in the sky—red to white to red to white—that mesmerized me. By the driver's own account, he lost control of his pickup while trying to get his puppy disentangled from his feet. I parked my vehicle on the eastbound shoulder of the road and somehow made my way across two lanes of freeway traffic on foot. I found the driver conscious. His upper body was trapped in the passenger compartment of the vehicle, his hip area was stuck in the rear window frame, and his legs lay in the cargo bed of the truck. The pickup itself was resting on its roof. I reached him from the tailgate of the truck by crawling through what felt like a tunnel. I discovered his femoral artery (located near his groin) was compressed in the mangled wreckage of the back window frame. The key was to slowly ease the pressure on his femoral artery, which I managed successfully. I'm not sure how long I was there before the paramedics showed up. I do remember we started to work closely as a team. The patient was disentangled from the vehicle with the help of the hydraulic wizardry of the jaws of life. (The dog was miraculously uninjured.) I travelled with the patient to the Kingston General Hospital, where I quickly became a target of merciless teasing. I had left Sunnybrook in my surgical greens, and coincidentally had just conducted a training session for emergency workers at the Kingston hospital a week or so before the accident. They knew I had a reputation for showing up at high-drama emergencies, and there I was, two hours out of the Toronto hospital where I practised, coming from a nearby accident scene dressed for action. Some of my colleagues still joke that I'm an accident waiting to happen, but it's nearer to the truth to say that if there is an accident, I'm likely to happen by.

I recognize now that my decision to live in a small room at Sunnybrook was telling. I would not be staying in Toronto. Canada's largest city was just one of those places "between my heart and home" in Nova Scotia, to steal a phrase from songwriter Kris Kristofferson.

Nova Scotia called in 1989 when Mike Murphy, the head of anesthesiology at Dalhousie University and the Victoria General Hospital, offered me a job in emergency medicine. I didn't hesitate to take the position. Mike gave me a warm welcome and even assigned me a small office space in which to store books and hang around. I soon made friends with Dr. Orlando Hung, a Hong Kong native who had just returned from Stanford after completing a two-year residency in anesthesiology. We quickly became close friends. Orlando was my kind of guy: inventive, curious, and innovative. He was qualified in anesthesia and had an advanced degree in pharmacology, and he was always looking for better ways to intubate patients and manage pain—particularly in children. Orlando and I began working on topical analgesics that could be applied to the skin—before giving a child a needle, for instance.

I also introduced him to a medical device I had worked on in my lab back in Pittsburgh. There, I had instructed Tudor Williams, a Calgary-based anesthesiologist, on using an adapted Flexi-lum surgical light (used in orthopedics) for tracheal intubation. Paul Berkebile, an anesthesiologist at another Pittsburgh hospital, had introduced me to the adapted orthopedic instrument. He had soldered a flexible wire to the surgical light. At the end of the wire, Paul had attached a small, high-intensity light bulb. Our own eureka moment came when we confirmed that the bulb transilluminated the route to the trachea (or windpipe) during intubation—essentially, you could see through the skin and steer the intubation tube easily through the glottis opening and into the trachea. Our new instrument had a flaw, however—one we discovered the hard way when our tiny navigational light bulb fell off and dropped into a patient's lung. Retrieving the bulb was easy enough. Fixing our new intubation instrument was a tough challenge, one over which I characteristically obsessed. Then I remembered that my dad, an innovative handyman himself, used a product called shrink wrap in his projects. When you heat shrink wrap, the plastic product holds virtually anything it wraps in a fierce grip. I went straight to a hardware store, bought a roll of shrink wrap, and used it to secure our light bulb to our adapted surgical light. It worked like a charm. Short of using small explosives, there was no dislodging the bulb from the end of the flexible wire.

My time as an inventor was short-lived. My mistake was writing the manufacturer (Concept Corporation of Clearwater, Florida) about the Flexi-lum surgical light and telling them about our innovation. I received no reply, but few months later I noticed an ad in a medical journal for the "new Tube-Stat intubating stylet." The corporation had essentially copied the design.[57] Frankly, I was too busy to care much, and resisted suggestions that we sue the company for pilfering our design. I was really striving to find a practical way for paramedics and others to intubate patients in the field or in any emergency setting. Use of an adapted surgical light was not ideal outside a controlled hospital setting, so I tested an old-fashioned way of finding the glottal opening—something I call digital tactile intubation. As the name suggests, the idea was to use your fingers to find the glottal opening by touch, and intubate the patient the same way. (Most adult fingers are long enough to perform this task.) Working with residents, we practised this on cadavers before using it in the field. It worked, and I eventually published a research paper on our findings.[58]

Back to Halifax in the late 1980s. Orlando was happy to use the adapted surgical light in his practice, and to tinker with the design. He was both a great clinician and a savvy entrepreneur and has patented several devices in his career. While Orlando and I were sharing a cramped office in Halifax, my old friend Geoff Garth showed up in Halifax. Geoff, the Long Beach surfer dude and former Mattel toy designer, immediately hit it off with Orlando. No surprise to me. They were kindred creative spirits. Geoff had founded one of the most innovative medical design and manufacturing companies in the world. (California Medical Products was incorporated in 1981; Geoff sold it to a Norwegian firm in 1991). In Halifax, Geoff and Orlando got lost in their world, and I began contemplating a complete change of direction—running for political office.

In politics, I soon learned, name recognition is an important asset. I'd earned mine the hard way in the late 1980s when my knack for landing in the middle of emergencies put me on the front page of the *Halifax Chronicle Herald* under the headline "Doctor Helps Avert Disaster."[59] The almost-disaster occurred on June 1, 1989, during a visit home, when I accompanied my parents to a church service. A new minister, Rev. Richard Robinson, was being ordained at Knox Presbyterian Church in tiny, beautiful Ross Ferry, Cape Breton. As we walked into the service, I immediately noticed the floorboards were trembling beneath our feet in the packed church. The floor collapsed quickly, raining floor timbers and well-polished floorboards down onto the Presbyterian elders gathered in fervent prayer in the room below. That's when my training kicked in, along with the understanding of building structure I had learned while following my dad around to odd jobs as a boy. I asked the congregants to exit the building in an orderly fashion by helping each other and tracking a route close to the exterior walls of the church, where I knew the floorboards would be best supported. I was frankly amazed, then and now, by how calmly the members of the congregation departed what was left of the building. (Maybe there's something to be said for Celtic stoicism, after all.)

Meanwhile, I clawed my way across what remained of the floor to the stairs leading to the basement, where I suspected the most seriously injured would be found. As I crawled through the rubble I came upon an octogenarian Gaelic-speaking friend, Malcolm Angus MacLeod. He was bathed in dust and debris, but when I greeted him in Gaelic (I knew only a few words), he raised his head and said, "Well hello, Dr. Ron—I guess the tea will be late tonight." I directed him to the exit. No one died in the incident, though several people were seriously injured. It was a pretty easy triage, overall.

Call it serendipity if you like—the next day, I flew to San Francisco to deliver a talk on "Aspects of Rural Disaster." I certainly had some fresh material to present. When I arrived at the hotel, one of my former residents, then a very active member of the emergency faculty at the University of Chicago, was delighted to see I was okay. "I just heard you being interviewed about your church collapsing last night!" she said. She was a faithful listener to *As It Happens,* a fixture of Canadian Broadcasting Corporation (CBC) programming. (It is broadcast in the US on numerous public radio stations, primarily NPR affiliates.) By the time I took the podium, the delegates had heard all about the church collapse, and the incident became the chief focus of my talk— and gossip around the conference halls.

The Ross Ferry incident, however, did not generate the kind of name recognition I would need as I contemplated a run at political office. Perhaps it should have forewarned me that I was about to face a series of crises of the political sort. Regardless, I had determined to paint on another large canvas by entering politics and working to modernize a healthcare system that badly needed it.

My interest in politics had been bred in the bone. I grew up in Cape Breton, after all, a place where politics is still described as either a blood sport or a religion. My own home became a quieter place— but not a more peaceful one—during election campaigns. My father came from a long line of Liberals, and my mom's people were staunch Tories—thus the uneasy truce as voting day approached. In a town where everyone talked politics all the time, my parents honoured a mutual vow of silence. I'm talking here about two people who never raised their voices to one another or to my sister or to me. Silence was as close as they would ever get to a declaration of disagreement. Until recently, in rural Nova Scotia, offspring traditionally voted for the same party as their parents. That left me in a curiously neutral position on politics as a child—and probably transformed me into a less zealous partisan as an adult.

When I was growing up, voters in my area chose between Canada's two mainstream parties—either the Liberals (the "Grits") or the Progressive Conservatives (the PCs or "Tories"). Not so long ago, vote-buying was the norm. Gifts were routinely handed out by party officials—pantyhose for the women, a pint of rum for the men—until at least the 1980s. In 1988, Harold Huskilson—a Liberal warhorse who also owned a funeral home on the province's South Shore—was linked to a vote-buying scandal after rum bottles were found stored in coffins on the premises in the run-up to the provincial election. Five of Huskilson's workers were later convicted on vote-buying charges.[60]

In my medical career, I had gradually come to the realization there were areas in the system that needed to change. At the same time, I felt that I had sort of abandoned my home province, so I began to look for a way to make a contribution. I decided I would have to get personally involved in order to make changes in healthcare. Then it hit me—I would have to get involved in politics in order to make the changes I thought were needed.[61]

By 1990 or so, I had decided to seek the Liberal nomination in the riding of Cape Breton North, which included my hometown of Sydney Mines. The timing should have been auspicious. The incumbent Member of the Legislative Assembly (MLA) for my riding, Brian Young (a Tory), was seasoned and skilled. Young had won three straight elections dating back to 1981, but he was showing signs of fatigue, as was the government he represented. Young's party had won power in 1978 under "Honest John" Buchanan, a consummate retail politician who never forgot a name and never ran out of steam. Even Premier Buchanan's friends might have conceded he was better at campaigning that he was at governing. But after he won his fourth successive election (against all odds) in 1988, his government started to fray at the edges. As political scientist Ian Stewart put it, "The final years of Buchanan's premiership seemed to epitomize the anachronistic quality of the traditional model of party government."[62] As his tenure ran down, one cabinet minister was found guilty of corrupt electoral practices, a few MLAs were caught up in expense account scandals, and two MLAs were caught breaching the confidentiality rights of citizens.

When I'd started to get involved in the Liberal party, around 1989, the tired Tory government should have been ripe for the picking— or more than ripe; the fruit was already rotten and falling off the branches. Unfortunately, the Grits' own orchard was anything but pest- free. The party had yet to free itself of a controversy involving kickbacks from government liquor store sales in the 1970s, when the

Liberals had last been in power.[63] In a practice known as tollgating, booze merchants paid a fee to the party for every case of product sold to the Nova Scotia Liquor Commission (all liquor was, and largely still is, sold through stores regulated and run by a provincial Crown Corporation). Between 1970 and 1978, the Liberal party raked in more than $4 million from illegal kickbacks—a lot of money in that era of politics, especially in a tiny Canadian province of fewer than one million people. Journalists and Opposition politicians feasted on this story, which featured a trio of colourful bagmen, one of them nicknamed "Suitcase" Simpson. (You needed a bag to carry all that cash around, after all.) The party's second mistake was not giving the illegally raised money to a charity as soon as the scandal was uncovered. The lingering and justified media attention continued to undermine the credibility of the Liberal party as it prepared to run on a reform-minded election platform.

As a recovering Calvinist raised by teetotalers, I had watched this story, mouth agape, from the fringes of the Liberal party. I had to get my bearings as I prepared to formally offer for the Liberals and enter the strange, strange world of Nova Scotia politics. Vince MacLean, the besieged leader of the day, was under intense pressure to resign his seat after failing to defeat the seemingly vulnerable Conservatives in the 1988 general election. The anti-MacLean faction was based largely in Halifax and was directed against a leader with a strong power base in Cape Breton, where I intended to run. I was caught in the middle and wanted to stay there. As a "promising newcomer" on the fringes of the party—or "fresh meat" to throw into battle, if you prefer—I tried to stay neutral as a leadership battle simmered and then boiled inside party ranks. Politics felt like a perilous business to me, and I didn't want to get wounded in the crossfire before I had even started campaigning. The sometime clandestine, sometime open campaign to replace MacLean was led mostly by Liberals from Halifax—the provincial capital located at some distance from the leader's power base on my home island of Cape Breton. I was caught in the middle and struggled to stay on the sidelines. (It helped that, as a rookie politician, I had little power or influence.) In 1992, Vince gave up the battle and resigned.

In the wake of MacLean's resignation as leader of our party, a Welsh-born physician named John Savage won the leadership of the Liberal party of Nova Scotia, but only after a long and agonizing 1992 convention that started on June 6 and ended on June 20.[64] The cause of the delay was the evolving and untested "tele-voting" technology. The party had introduced voting by touch-tone telephone to enfranchise thousands of people. (Traditionally, party leaders were chosen in Canada by the few hundred or few thousand people chosen to attend a delegated leadership convention.) The tele-voting system was supposed to be an example of participatory democracy in action. The only problem was that the technology itself acted up. The computerized counting system bogged down and finally crashed under the deluge of call-in voters on June 6. This left a few hundred disgruntled voters on the floor of the convention and thousands of Nova Scotians at home dazed and confused.

It also left the two main contenders waiting for two weeks to see who had won the job. The protracted vote cast Don Downe, a chicken farmer who favoured French cuffs and looked to some like a city slicker, against Savage, who hailed from the city and looked to some like a chicken farmer.

Savage, bearded and long-haired when he'd first emigrated from Wales in 1967, quickly became known as the "hippie doctor" in his adopted city of Dartmouth. He was my kind of physician. He started a program to help drug addicts; supported sex education programs in the schools despite the opposition of the Catholic hierarchy; and opened a medical clinic in East Preston, an African Nova Scotian community on the outskirts of Dartmouth.[65] On June 20, I was anxiously awaiting the results at a world heart association conference in Norway, which I had been invited to attend. At a formal dinner that evening (Norway time), my Norwegian hosts announced the results—that Savage had won the leadership—to the crowd, who by that time were well lubricated. They lustily cheered the result—not one of them knowing what the heck was going on.

In 1991, I had secured the Liberal party nomination in Cape Breton North by acclamation and was campaigning my shoes off in a door-to-door canvass of the riding. The uncontested nomination would have been a bit of a bore except that my mom, a lifelong supporter of the other party, showed up. Her declaration of loyalty to her son was somewhat ambiguous, however. She was wearing a dress so blue and bright it would have put a perfect summer sky to shame. Blue is the Tory (Conservative) colour in Canada. The Grit (Liberal) colour is red. On that night, my mom flew a blue flag in a red zone. She was supporting her son, all right, but she was not flying his party's colours.

Did I run a campaign that was a tad too eager? Looking back, I think I did. I even managed to secure a proxy vote from a lifelong Tory after I had treated him. His name was John Lamond, the uncle of my childhood friend Betty Anne. I had made my way home after a long day of campaigning when I got a call from Betty Anne, a registered nurse. Uncle Johnny's colour was off, she said, and he was refusing to go to hospital or otherwise get help. "But he'll let you see him," she said. When I got to the house in Sydney Mines, I could tell from across the room that Johnny was at death's door with congestive heart failure. I launched an earnest appeal to let me take him to hospital in the passenger seat of my Volvo station wagon. He agreed, with Betty sitting behind him in the old jalopy. It was a typical spring night in our corner of Cape Breton—wet, windy, foggy, and dark. At one point, as we drove along a winding coastal road toward to the hospital, I could tell Johnny was in trouble. Betty Anne managed to tilt his seat back, lean over it, and perform mouth to mouth resuscitation while I did my best to compress his chest with my right hand while driving with my left. We got him to hospital, the on-call doc intubated and admitted Johnny, and the man lived about a decade after that. I later went to visit Johnny in hospital, and during the visit he asked what he could do to repay me. I provided an answer that may have not strictly honoured the Hippocratic oath. "Give me your proxy vote," I said. I was being trailed by a group of nurses and docs during this visit, and they audibly gasped at my answer. (Candidates traditionally campaigned in rural hospitals and were usually accompanied by staff on their political rounds.) I never asked if Johnny's vote was cast on my side of the ballot, but I have a pretty good idea I lured him over to the Liberal side, if only for one election.

My campaign got a boost when I was appointed to President Bill Clinton's task force on emergency medicine in February 1993, just a few months before the provincial campaign. The story made page one of the local daily, the *Cape Breton Post*, which reported I was not only on the committee (true) but also its chair (false).[66] Alongside my campaign manager, Bob Jardine, and a growing group of faithful volunteers led by Jeff MacLeod (a political science student who seemed to work twenty-four hours a day and who was to become my executive assistant), I attacked the campaign with all the zeal I had brought to my crazed fundraising campaigns during my student days at Acadia. We knew cabinet minister Brian Young, my Tory opponent, had won the riding handily in the 1988 election. Poll-by-poll results from previous elections provided a very detailed understanding of voting patterns by street—and practically by household. I spent eighteen months on my feet, visiting every "PC" home at least three times and every "Liberal" home once or more. It was a clear strategy of keeping your friends close and your enemies—in my case, Tory friends and neighbours—closer.

The media feasted on just one political house call I made—or didn't make, as it turned out. In this case, I was so narrowly focussed on meeting a voter on the front steps that I knocked repeatedly on a door fronting a home that had burned down behind the entranceway. I persisted through an April blizzard until a neighbour's shouts, cutting through a howling wind, informed me, kindly, that no one was living in the charred remains of the building. (Yes, my ability to narrowly focus on a task can sometimes look like an eccentricity.)

In Sydney Mines I should have enjoyed a competitive advantage as a hometown boy who had made good and come back. Nothing could be further from the truth. Sydney Mines was a true-blue Tory town, staunchly Conservative and resolutely conservative. I tackled the challenge head-on by showing up on front doors almost as often as the milkman, and by painting Main Street Liberal red. North Sydney, the biggest municipality in the riding, was friendlier territory—so friendly that it was said the party could nominate a pig to run there and he'd sweep the town as long as he was spray-painted red. I suspect the operatives in the Liberal party, and the leader himself, thought I had little chance to carry the day on May 25, 1993. We had done our own polling, however, which showed we were probably winning. My team didn't really believe the results. (Our samples were small, our costs were low, our methodologies were suspect, and our analysis of the numbers was biased.) I decided to pull out all the stops. Win or lose, I figured I should leave some kind of legacy behind in my hometown, so I bought an old store on Main Street and renovated it as a campaign headquarters. We were enormously ostentatious about it all. Instead of calling our headquarters "Ron Stewart's campaign office," in the modest local tradition, we mounted a sign proclaiming the modest building to be the "Liberal Centre." We invited John Savage to the official opening of the building, and he actually showed up. Allan MacEachen, a Cape Breton political legend who had risen through the cabinet ranks to become the deputy prime minister of Canada, offered opening remarks. I couldn't have been prouder. MacEachen, who died in 2017 at the age of ninety-six, was one of the founders of medicare in Canada. He was also a champion, in his early years in federal politics, of higher wages for workers and pensions for Canadian seniors. Like John Savage, he was my kind of politician.

MacEachen and Savage gave our campaign a boost, but it was really led on the ground by a great local team, led by Jeff MacLeod, the scion of a well-known Liberal family and a young man who was to play a prominent role in my life in politics before writing his doctoral thesis related to healthcare reform in Nova Scotia. (Today, Jeff is a professor of political science at Mount Saint Vincent University in Halifax. He is also a talented visual artist.) We worked our butts off, and even managed to put a float in a parade in North Sydney. For that event, we recruited a crowd of young people, dressed them in sou'wester hats and rain gear, and equipped them with a temperamental fog machine that worked at the crucial moments. They waved to the crowd from our ridiculously long parade float that was decorated garishly in Liberal red bunting and featured a sign with a simple message displayed in huge letters: "Beaming through the Tory fog."

As voting day approached, we knew our campaign was gaining momentum for three reasons—support from the upper party ranks, our ability to bring young people into our camp, and the rather viscous campaign waged against us. A whisper campaign even alleged that I had refused to help a young person who'd needed medical care. The bogus allegation was endlessly repeated. I told my own team to ignore the innuendo and to offer no comment on the smear campaign. I wasn't about to breach medical ethics by speaking—for myself or through proxies—about anyone's medical condition. For the record, I should say I never for a moment believed that my main rival in the campaign was party to this personal attack. Election workers can be difficult to control, and their enthusiasm sometimes gets a bit overzealous.

On election day, my good friend Orlando Hung showed up at 7:30 A.M. He had made the long drive from Halifax in his big car, equipped with a satellite phone so we could keep in touch with headquarters as he chauffeured my workers around the riding. In the end, I'm not sure Orlando, with his nice car and fancier phone, was a vital part of my campaign effort, but I was sure glad to have his company on election day. There's no one with whom I would have more happily celebrated a victory. Perhaps more importantly, he was a reminder that I had a great job to return to in healthcare if the election went south that day. Every poll result I reviewed and every person I talked with told me I was winning the vote, but I still had the jitters.

My nervousness, it turns out, was unwarranted. I enjoyed the support of 5,459 voters. My main rival, Brian Young, garnered the support of 3,911 voters, down from more than 6,000 in the previous election. The voter turnout rate in my riding was almost 85 percent—almost an unimaginable number. We won easily, but I wasn't about to get all that excited about congratulating myself on election night. The night belonged more to John Savage than to his motley crew of candidates, many of them holding on firmly to his coattails. As a native of Wales, he became the first premier born outside of Nova Scotia—then a parochial province that was welcoming to tourists but not necessarily to newcomers. As a former hippie doc, and a former mayor who got away with using tax money to help developing countries obtain better water supply systems, Savage was an unlikely victor inside a small-*c* conservative province. He may not have been the first premier to run on a reform platform that included ending political patronage, but he was the first one who really meant it. Traditionally, government highway workers were fired en masse after power switched between parties in Nova Scotia. John Savage stopped that practice in its tracks, which surprised and shocked many Liberals.

The victorious Liberal caucus, including John Savage, would also have been wise to tell themselves on election night that while they owed their victory more to their leader than to the candidates, they also owed it more to history than to their leader. The Tories had also chosen a "reform" candidate—Donald Cameron—as their leader. Cameron, a former dairy farmer of fierce conviction, was (like me) a Presbyterian born and bred, and when he said he wanted to clean up Nova Scotia politics, he meant it. But as a veteran of the Buchanan cabinet, he was part of the old gang that history and voters were eager to sweep out of power after fifteen years. The Tories had grown tired, complacent, sclerotic, and corrupt in office. In our early months in power, we were idealistic, ambitious, energetic, and focussed. I was primed for action when I was sworn in as Nova Scotia's minister of health on June 11. My new job would land me in the strangest place I had yet encountered in my journey through life—the Nova Scotia legislature.

I was about to learn some bizarre lessons in democracy and how it works, starting with the realization that some of my closest allies in my effort to modernize the healthcare system would be found on the Opposition benches.

CHAPTER 9

FACING BRICKBATS AND FOILING BOOKMAKERS, 1993–1997

PREMIER JOHN SAVAGE'S GOVERNMENT LOOKED AS SAFE AS CHURCH ON JUNE 11, 1993, the day I was sworn in as the province's minister of health. Savage's Liberals held a clear majority; his cabinet was strong; his reform agenda was clear; and his ministers hit the ground running. My own goals as health minister were laid out on September 13, 1993, in the Speech from the Throne, which is the parliamentary equivalent to the US State of the Union address.

The Speech outlined our main priorities. Control and management of the healthcare system would be decentralized from the capital city, Halifax, to regional health authorities. A "seamless health system [would be] characterized by ready accessibility, woven throughout with the fabric of prevention, home care, acute intervention, and long-term care."[67] An "extramural hospital program" comprised of home-care services and community clinics would move the delivery services out of regional hospitals and into communities and homes. An emergency air ambulance service, as part of a "first-class emergency medical service" system would be put in place. We would wage war against Big Tobacco and win. Penalties for selling tobacco to minors would be increased; vending machine sales would be outlawed; and the minimum legal age for buying tobacco would be increased to nineteen from sixteen years of age.

Incredibly, we managed to implement many of these reforms in our first eighteen months in office, despite a lot of distracting background noise and a series of controversies—some of them real, some manufactured. Some of the barricades to reform were actually raised by my advisors in the civil service. Very early in my tenure as health minister I realized I also had to deal with something I will call the "Really, Minister?" syndrome inside the civil service. (This was a variation on "Yes, Minister," a phrase that seems to mean—inside the British civil service—that the Minister has been told his bidding will be done even though that's not about to happen.) The phrase "Really, Minister?" implied an unstated question, as in, "You can't possibly be serious, can you?" I got the "Really, Minister?" reply not once, but four times, when I kept instructing civil servants to end vending machine sales of cigarettes—that is, of the highly addictive drug nicotine, which is a killer. They eventually gave up on their passive but persistent resistance, and the ban made its way into law.

We thought our health reform package was boldly ambitious when it was launched; many critics would later describe it as naively audacious instead. In truth, we passed significant milestones in our first year in office, passing tough-on-tobacco legislation by the end of 1993, and introducing legislation to close rural hospitals that were virtually ungoverned and too often served as unofficial nursing homes.

On a personal level, I was saddened to see that my father was clearly fading into the dementia of Alzheimer's in the spring of 1993. (He would die that September.) The distraction of his disease helps explain why we all ignored a letter delivered to our family home from Rideau Hall, the home of the Governor General, Canada's head of state. My sister, Donalda Cavell, who had come home from Alberta to help with my dad and the election, eventually urged me to open the letter because it "looked important."

It was. I was being named to the Order of Canada, the nation's highest civilian honour. I got a bit of respite from the political wars in October of that year, when I travelled to Ottawa to be "invested" as an Officer of the Order.[68] I had invited my mom and Donalda to the ceremony. Donalda was the last of us to show up at our hotel suite in downtown Ottawa. I will never forget the first words she uttered after entering the room. Staring hard at my poor mom, who had put on her best going-to-church dress for the grand event in the nation's capital, Donalda said, "You're not wearing *that*, are you?" The dress, as I recall, was pale green and loose-fitting. It looked acceptable enough to me, but I knew I had to find a solution to our wardrobe woes the minute my sister pronounced judgment.

I thought of a way to reach family harmony. Earlier, I had spotted a fancy women's clothing store in the mall under the hotel, so I sent the two most important women in my life down in the elevator with my Visa card (hopefully not maxed out) in hand. It seemed like hours before they returned, bearing not only two new dresses but shoes to go with them. I'm not sure what outfit Donalda had intended to wear to the ceremony, but she clearly wasn't "wearing that" after sampling the quality alternatives. I recall the hotel suite saga more clearly than I remember the award ceremony on October 27, 1993, but I'm certain I was the worst dressed (in a well-worn tuxedo) of the three of us when Governor General Ray Hnatyshyn pinned the Order of Canada medal on my chest. Mom herself would scold me if I were to brag about the Order of Canada or other honours, but I was proud to be cited for "playing a significant role in the development of emergency medicine and ambulance care in Canada and abroad." I'm even prouder to say I was elevated to Companion of the Order of Canada (the highest level of the Order) on November 14, 2023. (Dozens of awards have come my way over the years, and while I respect every organization that bestowed them, the recovering Calvinist in me knows it would be unseemly to go on and on about them.)

An honest review of the first year of my political career has to highlight some high-profile controversies as well. By mid-October 1993, I was facing a call for my resignation.[69] By the end of the year, the *Cape Breton Post* (the local daily newspaper serving my constituency) was quoting anonymous sources within my own party questioning my performance.[70] On May 14, 1994, an angry crowd of an estimated seven hundred people showed up outside my constituency office in my hometown of Sydney Mines to demand the government slow down on its program to cut back on hospital beds and services in favour of putting community-based clinics in place around the province.[71]

On the same weekend as the protests, thieves broke into my home, ransacked it, and took everything I owned—from my stereo to my underwear.[72] (Fortunately, I didn't have much else to take.) To be clear, I never connected the break-in to the protestors who were trying to slow down our reform agenda. The thieves were clearly professionals, taking advantage of my presence at the rally to clean out the place in jig time. The protests that weekend got nastier still when my mother, then seventy-seven, became the victim of a cruel prank perpetrated by her neighbour in Sydney Mines. This gentleman, assuming wrongly that I lived in my mom's home, posted a sign on his property with an arrow pointing to hers. "Don't shoot," it read, "Ron Stewart lives next door." My mother came from tough stock, and Edith Cavell (MacLellan) Stewart was not easily rattled. But this prank devastated her. She didn't want to believe that people in her own community would treat her that way. I considered buying her an airline ticket to Calgary to spend some time with my sister, but she was not a woman to yield ground to a bully and she stayed put in her Cape Breton home.

Our government was stubbornly holding its ground as well, as a matter of principle. We had introduced far-reaching healthcare and economic policies, and we planned to see them through. During our tenure, regional economic development agencies were charged with spurring growth in rural areas of the province—areas that were struggling to hold onto jobs and young people. The province's dragon-sized deficit would be slain. The economy, slow to recover from the 1990 recession, would soar under a growth strategy that included tax incentives to entrepreneurs, grants and loans to leading industries, and the use of government procurement policies to build strength in the Nova Scotia economy.[73] (Such were our good intentions. Not all were realized.) Those policy initiatives, unveiled in the early months of our mandate, turned out to be a prelude to a series of pitched political battles that often impinged on my personal life.

There was no escaping this intersection of the personal and the political, as the circumstances surrounding my father's death will attest. In the last few months before he died on September 19, 1993, as Dad struggled through the last stages of Alzheimer's disease, my mother, my sister, and I tried and failed to get him admitted to the Sydney Mines long-term care facility, the Miners' Memorial Manor. The only option was admittance to an active-treatment bed in the Northside General Hospital in North Sydney. He didn't need hospital-style care at that stage; he needed end-of-life care. He didn't belong in the Northside General. Nor did the hundreds of other elderly Nova Scotians who were then warehoused in hospital beds, as they still are today, due to a shortage of nursing-home beds. My dad's situation was further complicated by a situation I was trying desperately to address as minister of health. As he lay dying, we were told that a bed might be "opening up" for him at the Miners' Memorial, but the bed was then occupied by an elderly man who was said to be routinely "dumped there" by his well-connected family when they went on holidays. My dad passed away in the hospital, where he shouldn't have been. I'd like to say this was an unusual situation in Nova Scotia, but it was anything but. Local hospitals and nursing homes were often scandalously used to provide free respite care for families with pull who wanted a break from looking after Mom or Dad.

On September 20, 1993, the day after Dad died, Premier Savage reached out to me. He apologized profusely for contacting me on the day the funeral service, but he had an urgent mission for me to complete. The premier asked me to visit the home of one Donald DeLeskie of Sydney. DeLeskie was staging a hunger strike while hosting a swarm of reporters from across Canada. DeLeskie had stopped eating in an effort to pressure the federal and provincial governments into conducting an epidemiological study of the impact of the Sydney tar ponds on the health of area residents. DeLeskie, a former steelworker from a well-respected Sydney family, had good reason to worry about the tar ponds, into which pollutants from the Sydney Steel Plant had been dumped for more than a century. (The plant operated from 1899 until 2001 under a series of owners.) The tar ponds were then described as the most toxic site in Canada, the dumping ground for an estimated 700,000 tonnes of industrial waste.

I went directly from the funeral to Donnie's residence. He lived in an old country-style house, and the room in which he held court was packed with journalists. With the cameras rolling and the tape recorders running, I told Donnie we didn't want him to get sick from a hunger strike. I said we'd do everything we could to clean up the tar ponds and would work with the federal government to fund an epidemiological study. I'll never forget his response. He said he guessed he would have to listen to any man who came straight from his father's wake to talk to him and agreed to end the hunger strike.[74] I remember driving away and thinking to myself, "How did I ever get into a job like this?"

My visit didn't mark the end of DeLeskie's campaign, which he waged alongside his twin brother, Ronnie, a quieter sort of activist. Donnie continued to push for a cleanup of the tar ponds and, in 1999, he attracted worldwide media attention by wading into the toxic brew himself. Wearing rubber boots and old clothes, with a spade in hand, he started to shovel out the gunk himself in hopes of speeding the cleanup along. A television reporter at the event, apparently overcome by fumes stirred up by Donnie's shovel, collapsed on the scene and was rushed to hospital—a made-for-TV moment that made Donnie's point with dramatic flair.[75]

By 2013, the tar ponds had been capped and transformed into a public space called Open Hearth Park. The DeLeskie brothers had both died by then, Donald in 2008 at the age of sixty-two and Ronald in 2003 at the age of fifty-seven. In November 2013, the cycling area inside the park was officially named the Don and Ron DeLeskie Bike Park in honour of the twin brothers who'd fought so long for the cleanup. I snuck into the event honouring the brothers, quietly taking a seat in the back row while local cabinet minister Geoff MacLellan presided. A member of the DeLeskie family also took the podium long enough to praise me for my role in helping out veterans of the steel plant. The speaker didn't know I was there, but my nearby seatmates did and broke into respectful, if not wild, applause. Seventeen years after leaving politics, it was still impossible for me to travel incognito on Cape Breton Island.

It was because of my visit to the DeLeskie home on the day of my father's funeral that my own name was mentioned in the debates of the Nova Scotia legislature on September 23, 1993. The speaker was John Holm, a member of the New Democratic Party. (The NDP, often called Canada's third party, are pure social democrats, with values similar to those held by left-wing parties in northern Europe. From an ideological point of view, the NDP would have been my party of choice—and I might have joined it if I'd thought it stood any chance of forming a government.) Holm praised me for showing "genuine compassion" to Donnie DeLeskie, "at a time when the minister himself was dealing with a personal family crisis."[76] I then rose in the House to praise my late father. "His was not a legacy of public acclaim or of awards," I said. "His was a legacy of hard work for forty-five years in the coal mines of Cape Breton, and his was a legacy that I pay tribute to in my work here in this House."[77] The occasion of those remarks was a sad one, but I welcomed the opportunity to commemorate my dad.

Here's one final story that connects my dad's life and death to my political career. As his health deteriorated, my mom, sister, and I discussed openly that the end was near and we should be prepared. We also decided it would be right to give his body to medical science. At about the same time, knowing of Dad's condition, I had approached my neurology colleagues at the medical school regarding the recent rumour that a Brain Research Centre was being opened at the school. I'd offered to back those efforts with the stamp of approval (and possibly funding) from my ministry, and things moved along fairly quickly toward their goal. After Dad's death I contacted those involved in the initiative and offered Dad's brain as one of the first donations to the centre. My colleagues assured me that this donation—as with all others—would be kept in strictest confidence.

In my first year in cabinet, I quickly recognized that the controversies generated in my own portfolio were often linked to the central paradox of the Savage government. John Savage led a parsimonious and prudent government run by lifelong progressives who would have preferred—in better economic times—to spend additional money on education, healthcare, and social services. In essence, the financial crisis facing the province had turned us all into reluctant fiscal conservatives. By 1993, that crisis was so severe that any government in power had to manage from the right—at least as far as spending was concerned.

The situation was so bad that the Conservative government that preceded us had ignored one of its primary duties before calling an election: bringing down a budget for the 1993–94 fiscal year. So bad that the Tory government had assessed its 1992–93 deficit at $132 million, while the credit rating agency Moody's pegged it at $641 million.[78] (Moody's was closer to the mark.) The great promise of the Savage election campaign, and the primary goal of the Savage government, was to take quick measures to stimulate the economy in the wake of the 1990 recession. Grow the economy, the thinking went, and government could generate enough revenue to support healthcare reform and other social policy measures. Fiscal policies, including spending cutbacks, were designed to secure the future of quality healthcare, education, and social services.

To say the least, fiscal matters are not my forte, and the dire financial straits facing our rookie government may provide some context for my own challenges in the health portfolio. Our government was determined to transform a massive deficit into a surplus within four years, while I was charged with introducing what turned out to be costly reforms in healthcare. Consider just one budget item: the cost of the government's home-care program, part of our effort to move treatment out of institutions and into communities, soared to $70 million in 1995 from $18 million in 1994.

Well before those numbers were put on the record in the legislature, I was a victim of unexpected events—that curse that inevitably afflicts governments new and old. As I mentioned earlier, I had only been in the health minister's job a few months when critics started demanding my resignation. In October 1993, NDP Leader Alexa McDonough called for my political decapitation after I publicly (and somewhat hesitantly) voiced support for the development of a blood fractionation plant in the suburban Halifax community of Bedford.[79] A strong argument could be made for building the plant in Canada, which depended on international supplies for 96 percent of fractionated blood products such as plasma. Canada was said to be "uniquely vulnerable" to foreign regulatory oversight of export blood products, international supply disruptions, and global price spikes.[80] In addition, the proposed Bedford plant would create four hundred knowledge-industry jobs in a poor province.

The argument for the plant seemed sound enough in theory, but its proponents (the Canadian Red Cross and the US biopharmaceutical giant Miles) were—to put it mildly—suspect in the public mind. Before we came to power, the Red Cross had distributed tainted blood products to thousands of Canadians (mostly in the 1980s), infecting them with what was then the deadly human immunodeficiency virus (HIV) and the hepatitis C virus. Red Cross bureaucrats were judged to have sacrificed the safety of the blood supply in a rush to meet demand.[81] The list of transgressions, later confirmed by a federal inquiry, was a long one. The shortlist included the following: untested blood was taken from high-risk donors; plasma was imported from US prisons and other suspect areas; and hemophiliacs received tainted blood products from inventory supplies as the Red Cross delayed purchasing safe heat-treated products.

By the time the federal commission of inquiry, under Justice Horace Krever, was announced in October 1993,[82] one Nova Scotia victim of tainted blood products was already a household name. Randy Conners, a hemophiliac, was a persuasive and compelling critic of the Red Cross. He had contracted AIDS from tainted blood in the mid-1980s, shortly after meeting his future wife, Janet. Randy was suffering from failing health by the time the Krever inquiry was called, and he died the following September at forty-eight years of age. Janet Conners, who also contracted AIDS and would die in 2022 at sixty-six years of age, was a powerful and passionate advocate who was rightly credited with forcing the federal government to call the Krever inquiry.[83] The Conners's recognition as folk heroes in Nova Scotia was secured by the time our party took power in 1993.

When our government supported development of a Red Cross-linked blood fractionation plant, the backlash came at us fast and furious. Alexa McDonough, the NDP leader, and I were soulmates on political matters and were destined to become close friends. But she didn't hesitate to call for my resignation not once but twice in October 1993, suggesting I was subjugating "health responsibilities to economic development considerations" by supporting development of a blood fractionation plant that would be operated by the Canadian Red Cross.[84] When I reviewed the press clippings from that month, I noted that my defence of the fractionation plant was lukewarm at best. I said the development had not attracted a penny of government support, and that the decision to build it belonged to the sponsors, not the Savage Liberals. "The Canadian Red Cross Society and its partner Miles Laboratories will build a plant somewhere and they have chosen Nova Scotia," I told the *Cape Breton Post*. "Now, whatever we may think of this decision, that is their right to do so."[85]

Why did my defence of the Red Cross plant sound less than passionate and full-throated?

Because I only half believed it.

I wasn't fully convinced the plant (which would never be built, by the way) was a good idea. As a citizen and a physician, I sympathized with Alexa's view that our government had allowed economic interests to trump healthcare concerns by supporting the plant. And in my gut and my brain, I wholeheartedly supported Janet Conners's argument that no decision on the fractionation plant should have been taken before the Krever inquiry issued its report (which didn't happen until 1997). As a cabinet minister, though, I was compelled to support government decisions regardless of my personal views, and I certainly understood the premier's view that we had to promote economic growth to keep the lights on. Politicos tell us the public solidarity of cabinet is one element of the discipline of power, which is so essential to effective parliamentary government. Rogue cabinet ministers can bring down a government faster than the most acidulous, or the most articulate, opposition critic. Still, this was a heck of a hard adjustment for me—working inside a cabinet that had to present a united front. I had been trained, nurtured, and steeped in the principles of medicine—and in my Calvinist heart I didn't stop believing for a minute that patients and public health always came first.

The tainted blood scandal—now, that was a genuine issue, as was our decision to support the fractionation plant. In that first year or so, I also found myself accused of committing every imaginable sin short of killing and burying union boss Jimmy Hoffa. In December of 1993, as I mentioned earlier, I was said to have lost touch with a riding I visited almost every weekend. In quick succession after that, over the course of the next year or so, Opposition critics said I was spending too much money on travel and meals. In truth I was and am parsimonious (perhaps to a fault) when it comes to dining out on my money or the taxpayers' dime. Champagne tastes? I don't normally drink the stuff, and aside from the occasional glass of wine with dinner, my lips rarely touched alcohol. My travel expenses were indeed higher than those of some of my fellow legislators, for the simple reason that my riding was more distant from Halifax than all but two or three of the province's fifty-two constituencies. (I was both blamed for not travelling to my riding and accused of spending too much money on travel.)

I didn't let the daily theatre of the legislature—where MLAs can utter any allegation they like without fear of legal consequences—bother me too much. Maybe I should have. I now recognized Opposition MLAs were effectively using their opportunities to ask me tough questions inside the legislature. Gradually, they mounted a strong argument that suggested I was taking specific services away from rural areas by closing some rural hospitals and moving some tertiary care to the city. In addition, they said our plan to transition to community- and clinic-based care in rural areas was neither well-thought out nor well-funded. People unfamiliar with the parliamentary system of government have little idea how punishing it can be for ministers and prime ministers. Often, I was compelled to answer fifteen or twenty probing questions per day in an open legislative, no-holds-barred debate. I still think this is the best system of government in the world. Ministers are elected directly by the people and are accountable to the public through Question Periods in the legislature.

Public protests were another challenge. Our healthcare reform agenda was wide-ranging and far-reaching, but I still had three priorities. One was tougher tobacco legislation; one was modernizing ambulatory, pre-hospital, and emergency care; the third—moving care out of regional hospitals and into community clinics and people's homes—seemed innocuous but proved the most controversial.

It was that issue that attracted seven hundred angry people to the street outside my constituency office on Saturday, May 14, 1994. I ignored the advice of political staffers by showing up at the rally rather than staying away and staying safe. (By this point in my tenure, I had reluctantly agreed to travel under police protection in Cape Breton, my home turf and the only area of the province in which this was deemed to be necessary.) In essence, our plan for rural hospitals was to close some and put the remainder under a new management structure that included some measure of control by the Department of Health, whose senior bureaucrats lived in faraway Halifax, not a universally beloved capital among rural Nova Scotians. Rural hospitals were then managed by local boards of directors, and they were highly politicized.

I faced that angry crowd outside my constituency office in Sydney Mines. The protestors had started gathering early that morning and would later march on both the nearby Harbour View Hospital and the Northside General. With local municipal politicians on hand and children in tow, they were primed to meet me but not greet me by the time I showed up. What I recall most vividly about that day is a vision of my two constituency assistants—Elizabeth (Tip) Thompson and Kim Rideout—forming a sort of palace guard outside my office on Main Street. With their arms folded over their chests and their gazes fixed, they were not about to let the "enemy" pass through the gates.

I knew, of course, that I was not there to talk to enemies but to friends and constituents, some of whom I had known my entire life.

The *Cape Breton Post* version of the story,[86] which I have no reason to doubt, says I tried to calm the crowd, saying our government would operate a healthcare system that provided hospital care in hospitals and primary care in more appropriate settings, including clinics. I also pointed out we had to reallocate funding to deliver more effective care—by shortening surgical wait times, for instance. A volley of insults and accusations were hurled back at me, the most common being I should return to the United States where I was said to belong.

One criticism that day came from a fellow physician, Dr. Wayne Bell, who said local people didn't know how care would be provided once hospitals were either closed or assigned new roles in the healthcare system. He told the *Post*, "There are no alternatives being put in place."[87] This criticism was commonly expressed, widely believed, and patently unfair. We had no intention of closing facilities like hospitals before alternatives were put in place. (Dr. Bell, I will add, came to the debate with his own agenda—he had run my Tory opponent's campaign in the 1993 election.) Our healthcare reform package had been published a year earlier during the election campaign, and the focus on community-based medicine was crystal clear.[88]

Still, in the highly charged politics of the day, people understandably feared losing what they had before a new care model was put in place. In addition, local hospitals, like local schools, were seen as part of the fabric of rural communities. I was to learn this the hard way as I toured the province in 1994 to explain the introduction of what we called our Quality Healthcare Initiative. A meeting in Berwick had to be cancelled due to security concerns. A year later, a second session in the Sydney area, this one focussed on our reforms to how doctors were compensated, turned into a near-donnybrook after Bruno Marcocchio, a veteran activist and a bit of local legend, started heckling me from one of the front rows of the meeting. At some point, I decided to talk directly to Bruno, a burly man whose voice could be heard a mile off in a howling Atlantic gale. He was nonplussed by the face-to-face conversation with me. First, he became quieter. Then he moved closer and closer to me, his face reddening. I don't remember feeling threatened, but Dr. Dan Reid read the situation differently. (I had retained Reid, who had served in Nova Scotia's cabinet in the 1970s, to help manage our government's testy relationship with Nova Scotia physicians.) As Reid remembers the story, he clutched Bruno from behind, first by one arm, then by the other, and marched him out of the meeting. Everyone got out of the event uninjured, but the evening could not be described as a shining example of how to win friends and influence people.

I can't say I had an easy time urging reform measures among my fellow physicians, either. In fairness, we did ask docs to accept a lot of change in a hurry. The battle unfolded on several fronts. We wanted to move non-tertiary (non-specialist) care out of hospitals and into community clinics and people's homes. Simply put, it cost way too much money to treat people in hospitals who could be helped in their homes or in clinics. To many doctors, these changes represented an attack on the comfortable status-quo arrangements under which patients went to see their family doctors in their offices. Suffice it to say that physicians were not eager to embrace change in the way they delivered care their patients. We also wanted to address a serious shortage of physicians in rural areas. To put it bluntly, there were too many family docs practising in the Halifax area and too few in the more remote parts of the province. Our solution was to offer financial incentives for doctors who would either relocate or set up practices outside the city. The Medical Society of Nova Scotia (now Doctors Nova Scotia), representing the province's physicians, fought me tooth and nail for two years as I restructured healthcare delivery and proposed major changes to the way docs were paid. Reforming the fee-for-service schedule riled my colleagues more than anything we proposed. I don't want to say the leadership at the medical society, and some of its members, had dollar signs in their eyes, but it sure felt that way at times. My medical school classmate, Dan Reid, later told one interviewer the Medical Society "preferred healthcare reform that goes slow, with no negative impact on their personal incomes."[89] Our government, on the other hand, was determined to introduce reforms in a hurry, while addressing an urgent need to trim spending. (And yes, we did trim the health department's budget allocation in the 1994–95 fiscal year.)

I was fifty-one years old by the time my argument with the Medical Society really heated up in 1994, but I was still too naive to anticipate the bitterness of the battle. I was also saddened by how personal it became. The Medical Society took out newspaper advertisements suggesting I couldn't be trusted to provide medical care in an emergency situation at 3:00 A.M. This was nonsense and the leadership at the society knew it. I was a rookie politician, and in some ways a rank amateur, but I had as much experience in emergency medicine as any physician then practising in Nova Scotia. (In the early 1990s, only six qualified emergency medicine specialists were practising in Nova Scotia.[90]) I don't know whether I laughed or cried when I read the list of reforms the Medical Society promoted in its infamous "three in the morning" ad.[91] The ad called for more rural docs; fewer physicians in over-serviced areas; more effective provision of healthcare in community clinics; and an expanded role for nurses and other health professionals. Wait a minute! That was our government reform agenda, and I believe to this day that if the Medical Society truly endorsed our policy goals, it would have worked with us and not against us. In retrospect, I see that the society was hitching its wagon to our policies because it suspected the ideas enjoyed public support.

The Medical Society wasn't the only organization that wanted my head brought into a banquet hall on a platter. Others, including opposition politicians, kept calling for my resignation. Premier John Savage—my soulmate in his belief in the need for reforms—kept rebuffing the critics. He was one tough politician, and I never doubted he had my back even when it would have been politically expedient to boot my posterior out the door. I may not have had a close personal relationship with John, but I couldn't have had a better political ally.

I also needed him.

✱

My struggles to reform healthcare were not focussed only on battles with doctors and with Big Tobacco and with Nova Scotians who wanted those rural hospitals kept open. I was also waging a war with the Ambulance Operators Association of Nova Scotia (AOANS).

This skirmish took me back to my early years in California when I recognized that some City of Los Angeles ambulance services were operated as profit centres by funeral home owners. In Nova Scotia, some attendants were trained—though not to high standards; others flew by the seat of their pants. I knew this from personal experience as an emergency doc in Nova Scotia. On Easter Sunday 1991, we treated a fifteen-year-old boy in the VG emergency department.[92] He had been found lying on a Halifax sidewalk. He was clinically dead upon arrival, with no detectable heartbeat. At the VG, we hooked him up to a defibrillator as someone started an IV. We gave the young man a jolt of electricity, which restarted his heart. Within minutes, he regained full consciousness, but he was one extraordinarily lucky lad. Had he suffered this catastrophe outside the city, the statistics showed he would have had a 1 percent chance of survival. Inside the city, where patients had better—but not great—access to emergency health services, his odds of surviving were only 10 percent. No element of the healthcare system needed urgent reform more than emergency services.

Fortunately, I was able to recruit the perfect ally in my effort to fix the system. I begged Mike Murphy, my former boss at the VG Hospital, to report on the state of ambulance services in Nova Scotia. Mike, who by 1993 was serving as the head of the emergency department at the IWK Hospital for Children, was ideal for the job. A qualified emergency physician and anesthetist, Mike suffered no fools and minced no words.

The so-called "Murphy Report"[93] zeroed in with pinpoint accuracy on the flaws in the existing ambulance service, which was basically a closed shop operated by members of the "politically and economically powerful" Ambulance Operators Association of Nova Scotia.[94] The organization's contract with government required operators to deliver "reasonable Ambulance Service," though no definition of reasonable was provided with regard to care.[95] Standards of care, medical charting requirements, response times—none of these was included in the AOANS contract with government. Under that contract, only AOANS members qualified for the financial assistance to carry patients. The operators also received more money, on a per-kilometre basis, for carrying corpses than breathing bodies. A separate contract for vehicle inspection was given to the AOANS. Essentially, one member of the club would inspect another member's ambulances. The training of attendants, also paid for by the provincial government, was essentially left in the hands of ambulance operators. Under this abysmal oversight system, some operators provided adequate emergency care to Nova Scotia, but none was compelled to do so by law. The Murphy Report noted that many operators in rural Nova Scotia were operated by multi-generational family businesses that ran funeral homes (or in at least one case, a gas station and taxi service) as an adjunct to the ambulance service (or vice versa). Murphy's report, written with co-author Ann Petley-Jones, describes the AOANS as a "poorly organized herd… operating in a non-coordinated, profit-driven system. The Department of Health acts as a bill payer with no evaluation process and without any medical accountability at all."[96]

Murphy was even more direct in interviews. When he spoke to Acadia student Jeffrey MacLeod for his MA thesis in political science, Murphy said, "Fundamentally [the ambulance service is] a transport service, a trucking system based on fee for service. It is operated with business objectives in mind with less emphasis on patient care issues. Even the Department of Health viewed it as such; there was no notion that this was a medical venture.… There is no medical accountability at all."[97]

Once Murphy had diagnosed the illness afflicting emergency services in Nova Scotia, he went on to identify a cure. His report recommended establishment of a professional Emergency Health Services agency operating at arm's-length from government. First responders would be better trained; at least one licensed emergency medical technician (EMT) would be part of an ambulance team of responders; a hospital paramedic program would be set up; ambulances would meet standards for highway safety while being equipped with the right medical equipment to save lives in the field; and an air ambulance service would be established. These were only the key recommendations inside a report that provided a blueprint for the establishment of a modern, effective EMS system in Nova Scotia.

I knew from the outset the controversy resulting from the Murphy Report would register high on the political Richter scale, and I still endorsed it without reservation in my role as minister of health. I had learned back in LA and Pittsburgh that plain English was just the ticket if your goal was to introduce significant or even radical change in the provision of emergency medical services. I also learned, from dealing with the legendary reporter Andy Schneider in Pittsburgh, that journalists can serve as allies in a good cause. Unlike many of my colleagues, my experience with journalists was a positive one. I always dealt directly with reporters and answered every question they asked to the best of my ability. What I got in return was fair treatment. That made me an outlier, but I was in politics to reform healthcare in Nova Scotia, not to win the next election. My hunch with regard to the Murphy Report was that it was certain to generate the right kind of headlines across Nova Scotia, and my hunch was right.

I did come to understand the views of private ambulance operators in rural Nova Scotia, though I thought they had no place in the health system over the long term. Robert Schaffner, the long-serving president of the AOANS, argued rural operators couldn't rely solely on the ambulance services to keep their businesses viable.[98] Ambulance services had to be operated alongside other businesses, most often funeral homes. Schaffner was also right to say the operators lived where they served, liked where they lived, and had to operate with some measure of professional competence just to walk down Main Street. But there was also a gap in the AOANS argument—one through which I was able to drive a fleet of modern, well-equipped ambulances staffed by trained attendants and paramedics. The association's mistake was insisting, repeatedly, that it was the role of government, not the operators, to establish and regulate standards of care in the ambulance sector. This was the AOANS's way of saying its members were not responsible for any shortcomings in the delivery of care, but it also allowed our government to say, in essence, "You're darned right it's our job to regulate standards of care, and we're going to do it."

To use the lingo of the public relations profession, Mike Murphy's report "prepared the market" for reform of emergency medical services, which became known as Emergency Health Services (EHS) in Nova Scotia. Murphy had publicly defined a problem that had to be solved. That gave us permission to tackle the issues—and again Murphy was key to getting the job done. He agreed to take a position on a contract basis and proceeded to help usher the enabling legislation through the provincial legislature.

It was a tough slog. The AOANS accused our government of proposing to introduce a costly "Cadillac" EHS system that would disrupt rather than improve emergency services in rural areas. Worse, I was said to be in favour of a "US-style" ambulance service. (Canadians cling—somewhat irrationally—to the view that their publicly funded, single-payer healthcare system is superior in every way to the American system, regardless of any evidence to the contrary.) In truth, though, we never intended to exclude private operators from delivering emergency health services in the province. AOANS members were free to submit proposals, under an open bidding system, for providing emergency services using well-equipped vehicles and trained professional responders.

This didn't stop the debate from getting extremely personal. My colleagues in the Liberal caucus were lobbied intensely. My personal integrity was questioned, and one old friend who operated an ambulance system went so far as to ambush me in the Sydney airport and repeatedly contact my aging mother with his complaints. One ambulance service owner also showed up unannounced at my offices in Sydney Mines and Halifax. He shared personal letters between himself and his wife underlining how financially ruinous EHS reform was to him personally.[99] Later, he took his complaints to media, sharing the result of a polygraph test he had taken as proof of the veracity of his allegations. He insisted my officials and I had told him, separately, that the department of health would extend financial support to him. I was more saddened by than angry about his accusation. He clearly overplayed his hand and lost credibility in doing so.

Despite all the sound and fury, Bill 96, the Emergency Health Services Agency Act, finally passed its third and final reading in the legislature on June 30, 1994, the year it was introduced. By 1996, we had used powers put in place under the act to put 150 new ambulances on the road and were ready to deploy medevac helicopters, a fixed-wing aircraft, and a critical care land ambulance transport unit. Most significantly, the bill gave cabinet the power to quickly introduce regulations that would define and establish professional care standards inside an ambulance system while working at arm's-length from government.

Reform of EHS was the crowning achievement of my life in politics. It's tempting to attribute this success to the fact that this was the field I best understood. But I know I couldn't have introduced a new EHS system without the support of Ann Petley-Jones and Mike Murphy, who in essence gave up years of his professional life to get the job done. Murphy was that rarest of characters in the drama of modern political life—he was an agent of change parachuted into a system of governance that usually defended the status quo. It's no accident that he was not a civil servant but a medical professional passionate about reforming a system he knew was badly flawed. Today, Nova Scotia's EHS system still faces challenges—paramedics feel underpaid and overworked, and they're right on both counts. In addition, they often end up stranded with ambulance patients for hours until understaffed emergency departments can take over the burden of care. This bottleneck ties up highly trained and highly committed paramedics, the type of professionals who gradually assumed their proper leadership roles in EHS as a result of our reforms in the 1990s.

I have to give myself mixed reviews for our other policy initiatives. We had promised, in our Throne speech, a seamless transition from hospital-based care to community-based care through home-care programs, small clinics in small towns, and a movement toward preventive health measures and health education. Tertiary or advanced care would be offered in bigger hospitals in bigger cities. Otherwise, the system would be decentralized. The boldest claim I could make in defence of our record in this area is still a modest one—we did establish regional boards, staff them, and start to introduce community-based care. But—and it's a big but—we encountered vociferous and sustained opposition to this initiative. Community leaders never understood why losing hospital services and advance care in their areas represented progress. In short, we had not defined a problem that needed to be solved. Instead, in the public mind, we were creating problems where none had existed. Political scientist James Bickerton sums up the problem pretty well in a single sentence in *The Savage Years*, which he co-authored: "Hospital and bed closures, salary roll-backs, layoffs, and pharmacare cuts dominated the news, while the new money allocated to setting up alternative home-care services and community-based programs was grossly inadequate."[100] Bickerton's comments point once more to our government's central paradox: We were progressive-policy liberals with too little money to spend on implementing the policies.

My battles with Big Tobacco started out well enough. By December 1993, six months after our cabinet was sworn in, we had passed my "Really, Minister?" legislation that banned vending machine cigarette sales, outlawed the sale of tobacco to people under nineteen years of age, and forced vendors to prominently display health warnings about tobacco products. It also imposed stiff penalties on vendors who sold tobacco illegally—$2,000 for a first offence, $5,000 for a second. This sounds like tame stuff today, but in 1993–94 I hosted delegations from several nations that wanted to know how we managed to pass such progressive anti-smoking legislation.

We also scored a victory of sorts by introducing smoking-cessation programs through the department. On the other side of the ledger, the government actually lowered tobacco taxes in early 1994. Cabinet made the decision while I was away in Cuba, and I was none too happy to hear the news upon return. Announcing the tax cut was a bitter pill, but I swallowed it on April 23 when I told the legislature that taxes would be lowered by seven dollars per carton in the face of massive black market sales of smuggled cigarettes.[101] This illegal trade in tobacco was a national problem, and most provinces joined the federal government in lowering taxes on smokes. "Unfortunately, the flood of cheap, illegal cigarettes into Nova Scotia has taken that deterrent from us," I told the legislature. "The government's ability to discourage smoking through taxation has been removed. We must, therefore, find new ways to protect Nova Scotians, particularly the youth, from tobacco addiction." I wish could have done more to curb tobacco use, starting with a ban on all advertising. I also regretted that my bill to ban smoking in the workplace and in other public places like bars and restaurants died on the order papers after I had left the minister's office. I wanted to do more. Heck, I would have liked to wipe the tobacco industry off the face of the earth, given the impact of their product on human health and happiness, and in light of what I'd seen of their lobbying tactics over the years.

In terms of my record as minister overall, I'd assign myself high marks for the emergency healthcare reforms, despite all the chaos that surrounded the initiative. We started to transition care to homes and communities from large institutions like hospitals, but this turned out to be a process—one that is still ongoing—and not an event. We were fast out of the gate with anti-smoking measures but could have done more on education and cessation programs. As for duelling with docs, the war to restructure the fee schedule was a nasty one, and I'm still saddened that the Medical Society of Nova Scotia launched an ad hominem attack on a minister of the Crown in paid newspaper advertisements, rather than doing its part to lower costs at a time when the province was in dire financial straits.

Looking back at our government's record, I can see that we promised too much too soon in the healthcare platform we announced during the 1993 election campaign. Our cabinet was made up largely of activists who worked to implement progressive agendas inside a province in which "don't-rock-the-boat" politicians thrived, prospered, and endured. One of our government's first austerity measures was the imposition of a 3 percent salary rollback on all civil servants making more than $25,000 per year. Doctors, who could vote with their feet by leaving the province, successfully fought against imposition of this measure in their ranks. Eventually, we did strike a new, more sensible fee agreement with physicians, which also allowed them to incorporate their businesses. Arguably, we put more money in their pockets while asking other public servants to accept less. On the plus side, we did create an incentive package (including a minimum salary for rural costs of $120,000 per year) that helped place more doctors in rural areas.

As for me, I never did become a political animal. I remained a product of the medical system in which we diagnosed problems on the basis of the best evidence and acted quickly on the basis of that evidence. In the political depths, I was a fish out of water, and I never really learned how to avoid the jaws of sharks. I now consider it a small miracle that we were able to take such giant steps forward by introducing a modern EHS system and passing progressive anti-tobacco legislation in the face of fierce lobbies. We also exceeded the expectations of the political bookmakers, pundits, and critics, who wrote us off as naive upstarts who would never beat the odds by introducing meaningful reform in healthcare.

On a personal level, my period in politics represented a prolonged dark night of the soul—or as close as I would come to one. And that's a heck of a confession for a recovering Calvinist. We're not much given to expressing our feelings. On an even more personal level, before I entered the political arena I had been all but immune to setbacks. Inside medicine, I could usually find a new way to achieve goals after something had gone awry. Inside politics, I found the partisan "warfare for warfare's sake" dispiriting, the internecine battles in the Liberal party disheartening, and the attempts to draw my aging mother into the political dramas intolerable. Eventually, the same party that chose John Savage as their leader after he promised to end political patronage dumped him (in 1997) for honouring that commitment.

I finally and gladly resigned my cabinet portfolio on June 20, 1996. Bickerton later called me an "unusual breed of cabinet minister, a mission politician" driven by "zeal for radical systemic reform."[102] There's something to that—I certainly felt like a fish out of water. In 1997, I found a way to gracefully exit the political arena altogether, vacating my seat so that the new leader of the Liberal party of Nova Scotia (Russell MacLellan) could run in Cape Breton North and gain a seat in the legislature. I am hardly a phoenix, but I was more than ready to rise from the ash heap of a provincial government and try my hand at global politics, where the stakes were higher and the politics were less personal.

CHAPTER 10

BATTLING BOMBS AND BUTTS,
1997–2017

GIANTS CAN SOMETIMES BE TOPPLED BY PUBLIC HEALTH ADVOCATES ARMED WITH NOTHING more than a slingshot and a sense of mission. And so it came to pass, on April 25, 1997, that the Tobacco Act (Bill C-71) received Royal Assent in Ottawa. The act, which banned advertising of tobacco products, made Canada the most progressive nation in the world in the battle against the poisons smokers inhale with every drag on a cigarette.

But the bill was a long time coming. Back in 1988, the Canadian Parliament had passed an act to ban tobacco advertising and phase out industry sponsorship of sporting and cultural events. In 1995, the Tobacco Products Control Act was struck down by the Supreme Court of Canada, which ruled it placed unconstitutional limits on freedom of expression.[103]

I claim only a foot soldier's part in this successful campaign, but the fight against tobacco was one of the most important battles of my life and career. Fortunately, a fellow Cape Bretoner eventually stepped into the breach. David Dingwall, a janitor's son from the tiny village of South Bar, was a protegé of two political legends—Jean Chrétien (then Canada's prime minister), and Allan MacEachen, the Cape Bretoner who had ushered in the country's first national medicare act in the 1960s.

Dingwall and I could not have been more different, and he managed to rub me the wrong way (to say the least) when he lobbied our provincial government in 1994 to lower tobacco taxes as one means of combatting cigarette smuggling. He was too aggressive, dogged, and relentlessly political for my taste. But those very qualities were needed to push his 1997 legislation through the Commons. Dingwall, who today is the president of Cape Breton University, served as Canada's minister of health for only eleven months, from July 1996 until June 1997—just long enough to perform a miracle, as it turned out. It's impossible to underestimate the odds stacked against Dingwall when he took over as minister of health.

As he told the story in a presentation to Dalhousie University's MacEachen Institute in 2017, the finance minister of the day, Paul Martin, was not overly pleased with the legislation.[104] Martin, who was destined to become Canada's next prime minister, headed a department that was determined to protect the significant tax revenues generated by tobacco sales. In civilian life, he had also been chair of the board at Imasco, the former owner of Imperial Tobacco. Martin and Chrétien both represented ridings in Quebec, the centre of the tobacco industry in Canada. Dingwall also knew, by the time his Tobacco Act was before the House, that Chrétien himself was wavering. He still decided to shoot the moon, introducing an ambitious bill, soon to be entrenched in law, which would both ban advertising and phase out event sponsorship by tobacco companies.

I resigned from cabinet in June 1996, quitting my job as Nova Scotia's minister of health six months after Dingwall was appointed to the same role in the federal government. But I was no shrinking violet in the battle against the tobacco industry, whether I was serving in politics or not. Dingwall later said he was grateful for my efforts to persuade other provincial ministers of health to support his tobacco legislation as he battled to bring his cabinet colleagues and the provinces to his side of the debate.[105] In early 1996, he wined and dined the provincial ministers in Ottawa in an attempt to recruit them as warriors in his anti-tobacco war. Many ministers were blasé about federal tobacco legislation—they had their own battles to fight back home, and there was little to be gained politically by helping Dingwall score a victory in Ottawa. I was always a physician first and a politician second, so I saw the issue differently. I knew tobacco was a scourge, particularly among young Canadians. This was no accident— the industry's business plan was founded on addicting teenagers, the younger the better. The earlier kids start smoking, the more likely they were to continue for the duration of their tragically shortened lives.[106]

On May 12, 1994, I stepped outside the lines in my role as provincial health minister by appearing before a House of Commons committee in Ottawa to support proposals to entrench plain packaging regulations for tobacco products in federal legislation. This was two days before the angry crowd of seven hundred Cape Bretoners marched on my constituency office in Sydney Mines to protest our government's plan to open community clinics and close some rural hospitals. A handful of critics inside Nova Scotia, including some fellow Liberals, thought I should stay close to home and look after politics and policy on my own turf, rather than put in what they characterized as a cameo appearance in Ottawa.

The critics were wrong. Tobacco was wreaking havoc on the health of Canadians (and continues to do so today), and there was no more important role for me than to fight Big Tobacco on a big stage. Furthermore, Prime Minister Jean Chrétien had promised to review plain packaging for tobacco products as part of his pitch when he'd persuaded Nova Scotia and other provinces to lower tobacco taxes. I was in Ottawa to fight for a true quid pro quo.

The tobacco industry had different ideas—it turned the "plain packaging hearings" into a high-noon shootout. As Rob Cunningham tells the story in his 1996 book, *Smoke & Mirrors: The Canadian Tobacco War*, the industry brought in some top guns from the US to wage its battle. Carla Hills, the former US trade representative under George H. W. Bush, focussed on trade law, not health impacts, in the evidence she placed before the committee. In a signed legal opinion, she said plain packaging of cigarettes would violate the terms of both the North American Free Trade Agreement (NAFTA), which she helped negotiate, and the General Agreement on Tariffs and Trade (GATT).[107] Her brief also argued that Canada would be required to compensate the tobacco industry under NAFTA rules if it introduced plain-packaging regulations. William Webb, the president of Philip Morris International, said in a letter that "if Canada adopts legislation in total disregard of internationally recognized trademark rights, this would be a significant consideration in any new investment decisions."[108] That was seen, rightly, as a threat to pull jobs out of Canada. Philip Morris and the companies it owned employed almost five thousand people in Canada at the time. (I'll say this much for Hills and her colleagues in the tobacco lobby—you couldn't accuse them of subtlety.)

In *Smoke & Mirrors*, Cunningham concludes that Big Tobacco overplayed its hand before the committee, and he cites then-serving federal health minister Diane Marleau in support of that view. "No US multinational tobacco manufacturer or its lobbyists are going to dictate health policy in this country," Marleau said.[109] Canadian media commentators were also critical of the tobacco lobby, which was called arrogant and said to "give corporate thuggery a bad name."[110] Despite the public outcry against the tobacco companies, health advocacy groups could not turn those 1994 hearings into a complete victory.

I was fifty-one years old when I appeared before the Commons committee; I was seventy-six years old in 2019, when the federal government of Canada finally introduced plain-packaging regulations. Thousands and thousands of Canadians died from smoking tobacco products in the intervening twenty-five years. Today, vaped tobacco products are generating huge profits for the tobacco industry, which continues to demonstrate the resilience, adaptability, and instinct for survival of a cockroach.

＊

I kept a journal during my political years and beyond (1993–98), and a couple of phrases ring true when I reread it today. I said my decision to enter politics represented "a change of direction" in my career, but not "a change of heart." I was determined to advance public health on a large scale, and that sense of mission kept me going through my hectic political years, when I was too busy to collapse in a heap of jelly, and after I left politics, when I felt dispirited enough to do just that. My journal tells me that the aftermath of politics left me with a fatigue "which penetrates the soul," as Pierre de Ronsard said. I suspect I was clinically depressed, as I had been during the years at Acadia University in the wake of the accidental death of my cousin Lawrence Stewart. And the remedy at Acadia in the 1960s was the same one I adopted three decades later in Halifax—I threw myself into action.

At Acadia, that had meant launching a bid to become president of the student council. In 1997–98, now free of politics, I charged off in several directions at once—working as an anti-landmines advocate, continuing to fight Big Tobacco, and educating students at Dalhousie medical school, where I also took on a job as director of humanities in medicine.

Well before I entered politics, I had been involved in the land mines issue as an executive member of the World Association for Emergency and Disaster Medicine (WADEM). WADEM has an odd history. It is a successor organization to something called The Club of Mainz, which was founded in 1976 by a leading group of physicians including the formidable Peter Safar, my colleague and mentor at the University of Pittsburgh. The goal of the original membership, initially limited to a hundred people, was to improve pre-hospital cardiac care across the world. As one commentator wryly put it, "We had men walking on the moon before we had advanced cardiac life support practiced in the streets here on earth."[111]

In September 1997, I introduced a motion at the WADEM annual meeting in Mainz to pass a resolution supporting the proposed United Nations Anti-Personnel Mine Ban Convention, the so-called Ottawa Treaty. It supported "the designation of such devices as cruel and inappropriate weapons of war."[112] This should have been an easy chore—no physician who has sworn the Hippocratic oath should be supportive of weapons of any kind. We were still worried that our members from China and Russia would balk at endorsing a treaty their nations were unlikely to support. In the end, the WADEM vote was unanimous in backing the 1997 land mines treaty known as the Convention on the Prohibition of the Use, Stockpiling, Production and Transfer of Anti-Personnel Mines and Their Destruction. Our colleagues from Russia and China were taciturn during the discussion of the resolution, and almost comically morose in their demeanour, but they did the right thing in the end.

I presented the WADEM resolution at a December 1997 meeting in Ottawa at which the Ottawa Treaty was finally signed. I was also named as the physician representative on the panel that discussed the impact of land-mine injuries on human beings. Despite the ongoing use of land mines, most notably in the current war between Russia and Ukraine, their deployment has been closely watched and regularly condemned since the Ottawa Treaty was signed.

Getting back into the wider world after politics put me in the company of like-minded people and old friends, but it also brought me face to face with the realities of growing older. I was entering that stage of life at which I attended more funerals than weddings, and I was saddened by the loss of several friends and colleagues. No one was closer to me than Thomas Michael (Mike) Moles, whom I had met during my LA years. Spy, raconteur, natty dresser, Moles was a legend in the world of trauma medicine, his expertise gained the hard way during five years with the Royal Army Medical Corps serving in Borneo and Nepal. In 1970, he created a major incident response plan that would become a "blueprint for many hospitals in the UK and abroad."[113] In 1980, he left England to take up a position at Hong Kong University, where he quickly became a leader in pre-hospital emergency response. Moles saw that first responders faced two major logistics problems in the city—traffic gridlock and a skyline filled with skyscrapers served by elevators too small for a stretcher. The solution to the first problem came quickly to Moles—put paramedics on motorcycles, a favoured Asian mode of transportation. His "motorcycle medics" soon became famous in the city, creating a model of first-response healthcare that was soon adopted in London, Australia, and several US cities. I worked with him for years trying to find a solution to the second Hong Kong challenge—how to treat cardiac patients on the upper reaches of high rises. It wasn't until the mid-1990s that this problem was partially addressed with the invention of the automated defibrillator, an easy-to-use portable device that can now be found in hockey rinks, grocery stores, schools, theatres, and other venues all over the world.

Moles would often invite me to lecture in Hong Kong, never more memorably than in 1997. That year, in the months leading up to the city's reunification with China, I met him at one of his favourite haunts, the infamous Foreign Correspondents' Club. (The club was portrayed in one John le Carré novel as a nest of spies.[114]) Moles, who smoked all day and could drink all night, made no secret of his second life as a member of the Special Services of the British Reserve Forces. He never discussed the details of his intelligence work, but when he was about to disappear into the ether he'd tell his friends he was away "paddling up the Amazon." While we were in the Correspondents' Club on the day in question, Moles said he was waiting for an unnamed man to deliver what he called important papers. Eventually, a mysterious figure showed up just long enough to drop a plain brown envelope on the table between us. The papers inside gave Moles the freedom to stay in Hong Kong after reunification with China in 1997. Mike did just that, remaining in the former outpost of the British Empire for four more years. He continued living with his partner, Pat Elliott Shircore, in a small village on the South China Sea. He always seemed indestructible to me, and I assumed he would smoke and drink his way into his nineties. Sadly, he died at home in 2001 at the age of sixty-six, after telling his partner he had just suffered a ruptured aortic aneurysm and would be gone within minutes. His final diagnosis was an accurate one.

Moles's death was one of many that gave me intimations of mortality in the early years of the new millennium. His old friend and colleague Peter Baskett, another inveterate smoker, was a sort of patrician version of Moles. I was able to reconnect with him as well through WADEM and what I call the international circuit of medical conferences. Alas, Baskett was also destined to die too soon, in 2008 at the age of seventy-three. Baskett, born the son of a peer of the realm, had what the *Guardian* called a "profound influence on the development of pre-hospital care in Britain and on the practice of resuscitation medicine worldwide."[115] In the late 1960s, he managed to persuade the Gloucestershire ambulance service to train attendants to administer pain relief analgesics in the field. Moles and Baskett, fast friends who were both brilliant public speakers, travelled the global conference circuit together for decades, with me playing the role of awestruck sidekick. (I enjoyed taking the podium myself, but following either of these gentlemen to the microphone was not for the faint of heart.) My old colleague Peter Safar, thrice nominated for the Nobel Prize in medicine, had survived the Holocaust and the lesser perils of Pittsburgh politics, but cancer took him away as well on September 13, 2003. He, too, had been a leader (and founder) of WADEM, a persuasive ally in its effort to rid the world of land mines.

I did my best to honour my colleagues' legacies by advancing work I had shared with them. In 2005, WADEM endorsed the Nairobi

Declaration and Action Plan on land mines, passed a year earlier at the first UN conference to review the 1997 Ottawa Treaty.[116] The Nairobi declaration endorsed the "unwavering commitment [of treaty signatories] to achieving the goal of a world free of antipersonnel mines, in which there will be zero new victims." If that was the goal from 30,000 feet, the underlying motive back here on earth was persuading non-signatory nations to endorse the Ottawa Treaty, most importantly the United States, China, and Russia.

Would a universal ban on land mines really deal with the problem? That question seized my imagination, so I put my research hat on and went to work in the archives. One problem with international weapons agreements, including the Ottawa Treaty, was that they focussed on a specific weapon rather than the effect such weapons have on the human body. In 1868, the St. Petersburg Declaration banned the exploding bullet, which seemed like a good idea at the time. Subsequent history still poses a crucial question about that declaration: "So what?"

The exploding bullet, as I explained in a 1998 paper, "Anti-Personnel Landmines: The Next Bold Step..." published in *Prehospital and Disaster Medicine*, was soon replaced by "high velocity missiles that produced far more terrible wounds."[117] In 1995, laser weapons that could blind an enemy were outlawed. A greater good would have been served by banning any weapons with the capability of blinding other human beings. That article seems like heady stuff, even egg-heady stuff for a guy who had spent so much of his life in the trenches of medicine and politics. But I was determined to play a role—albeit a small one—in public health writ large.

The death of John Savage, the hippie-doctor-turned-premier, hit me as hard as the passings of Moles, Safar, and Baskett. Each of the four men drew their last breath in that first decade of the new millennium, Savage on May 13, 2003, at seventy years of age. Savage was not as close a personal friend to me as Moles or Baskett, but no one had paid a steeper price for supporting me through a challenging period of my life. He had taken no shortage of advice from people—within our own party—who thought it would be expedient to fire me for the good of the party. Savage resisted their entreaties. Our alliance was born of a shared sense of mission—we were determined to reform Nova Scotia's healthcare system, and while we didn't accomplish half as much as we would have liked in those tough years, we did usher in twice as many reforms as the armchair pundits predicted.

The public reaction to his death said much about my native province. The story commanded the front pages of the province's daily newspapers. The *Chronicle Herald*, the province's largest and most influential newspaper, ran several stories under laudatory head-lines.[118] Savage was praised as an innovative, bold leader who brought in far-reaching reforms in healthcare and municipal government. Politicians of all stripes lined up to pay tribute to the man. In short, the same media and political establishments that gave him the bum's rush in 1997 when they forced him out of office gave him a hero's farewell in 2003 when he died.

In looking back on what followed the death of "my premier," I can at least take comfort from the tribute written by Mary Jane Hampton, a healthcare consultant, just days before he died.

> *Criticism at public meetings and from the Opposition benches about hospital closures and the lack of community programs was muted only by criticism from our own department of finance about the spiralling cost of delivering healthcare. There were days that felt pretty lonely. In the end, however, the healthcare reform agenda endured. A platform was created that made it possible for future governments to continue to implement the changes that everyone knew were necessary, but that few were prepared to risk everything to address. Thankfully, John Savage risked everything.[119]*

*

I travelled the globe more or less constantly in the late 1990s and over the first seventeen years or so of the twenty-first century. I was a seasoned speaker on the international medical conference circuit, if not a particularly predictable or polished one, and the conference agenda kept me in the air and on the road.

My reputation for quirkiness certainly preceded me; it could be dated to the delivery of one keynote address at which I managed to broadcast my performance not only from the podium but from the bathroom as well. This misadventure took place at a meeting of the National Association of EMS Physicians (NAEMSP). Forgetting that I was wearing a lapel microphone, I retreated to the toilet for a pre-speech pee, which was clearly broadcast to the audience, along with the sounds of my inevitable humming and mandatory handwashing. When I got back to the stage, I was greeted by an uproarious standing ovation, the first and, I'm happy to say, only time I endured such a rapturous reception before I was able to utter a single word of wisdom to the assembled multitude. (Years earlier, when NAEMSP was formed in 1984, I was elected its first president at the association's inaugural meeting, attended by a handful of physicians. My colleagues nominated and elected me as their leader—and designated drudge—while I was taking a bathroom break. My term in the leadership job became known as the "bladder presidency." As always, there is an important subtext to the humorous story; we formed the association to give a voice to our nascent field of emergency medicine.

I also travelled the world with two corporate leaders—Keith Condon of Tri-Star Industries, a Nova Scotia–based ambulance maker, and Geoff Garth, the toy designer who founded California Medical Products. I didn't take a penny in income for supporting the marketing efforts of the two firms. I took on the job of holding workshops for medical professionals with the intent of improving the designs of their products. Garth really did design a better cervical collar for emergency patients, as well as several other medical devices, but they worked only if people on the front lines knew how to use these tools. Teaching them to do so was my job. I played a similar role with Condon, whose company custom-designed ambulances for countries from the Middle East to the Caribbean. I travelled with Condon to teach paramedics how to best use the ambulances and equipment designed for use in their countries.

I also roamed the world, improbably enough, as a choirmaster and concert impresario, thanks to my appointment as director of the Music in Medicine program at Dalhousie University, and then as the director of the medical humanities program. I had big shoes to fill in this job, as the successor to Thomas John (Jock) Murray, one of the most remarkable and accomplished men I met in my sixty or so years in medicine. Murray, a Nova Scotian, was a global leader in the field of multiple sclerosis research and treatment.[120] He became a medical historian without peer, using his extraordinary diagnostic skills to probe some very cold cases indeed—including the illnesses and death of Mozart. Murray co-authored a biography of Charles Tupper, the Nova Scotia–born physician who served briefly as Canada's prime minister in 1896. Murray became the only non-American to serve as the chairman of the Board of Governors for the American College of Physicians. In his role as Dalhousie's dean of medicine between 1985 and 1992, he established what has been called a "world-respected program in medical humanities."[121] One of Murray's core beliefs held that physicians need to understand human beings and human values to be good at their jobs, a view I had held since transitioning from arts to sciences during my years at Acadia University.

As the faculty member charged with introducing medical students to the arts, my focus was on music. I formed a large cadre of mixed choral singers, with smaller groups to make touring easier. The men's singing group (the Testostertones) became popular and played to packed houses in the Maritimes and beyond in 2004. We raised some money for the program and had some fun touring around in a van acquired specifically for the epic adventure. I recruited talented singers from the community to join our medical school choir and led various groups on several tours of Southern California, calling on old friends to billet our musicians, often in the small surfer-style, beach community homes that many paramedics in the area preferred. We also made it back to my old haunts at the University of Pittsburgh, to Washington, DC, to several Ivy League universities, and to New Zealand for a national tour. We travelled, for the most part, on my credit card, leaving me stuck with debts I eventually paid off by fundraising and ticket sales.

These magical musical mystery tours sound as if they were a lot of fun and a lot of work, and they were—both. The Humanities in Medicine program was something else as well—a vital part of the medical education of my charges. The program's primary goal was to introduce the kind of work–life balance that docs so often urge on their patients. In addition, if you perform music on a ward in a hospital, or in a common room at a nursing home, or to an overworked group of medical professionals in a staff lounge, you can see shoulders relax and sense spirits lifting in the audience.

I clearly remember taking a small group of string musicians, brass players, and singers to the Northwood continuing care facility in Halifax, where we set up a pre-Christmas concert in the pub. Residents shuffled into the room leaning on their walkers; others were pushed there in wheelchairs with their heads bowed in what seemed to be silent prayer; some meandered in on their own steam. By the time we were halfway through our second Christmas song, heads were raised and eyes were focussed; feet were tapping to the music; and one couple rose from the couch to dance a duet to celebrate what I took to be a long and happy partnership. Music is not always the best medicine—sometime a patient in severe pain needs an opioid, not an opus—but music and theatre and literature certainly enrich the human spirit. As for the medical students I took along to that Northwood concert, they learned something from that appreciative audience that is too often lost in the grind of daily medical practice: every person they encountered was a human being with human needs and wishes and dreams. As Arthur Stairs had told me in my first year at medical school, that's a lesson I should never forget.

Throughout my life, my mom was my mentor and unbending support. When I was growing up in Sydney Mines, she did her best to teach me lessons in humility and humanity. When Anita MacDowell had finished at the top of our high school class, Mom told me to celebrate her success instead of getting into a state of high dudgeon about finishing in second place. When a dinner was held in my honour to mark my contribution to the emergency medical system in LA, she and my father showed up to mark the occasion—and, I expect, to remind me where I came from. When I ran for political office, she stuffed envelopes and knocked on doors, even though she, a lifelong Conservative, was doing so in support of a Liberal candidate. When I was named to the Order of Canada, Mom showed up in Ottawa for the ceremony alongside my sister.

She was behind me every day of my life, until one day she wasn't there anymore. She died on March 30, 2015, in her ninety-ninth year, in the palliative care unit at the Cape Breton Regional Hospital in Sydney. My sister and I were at her side. A lifelong Christian who took her faith seriously, Edith Cavell (MacLellan) Stewart had volunteered for everything from missionary societies to food banks while serving for longer than fifty years on the Harbour View Hospital Auxiliary. She forged a special bond with paramedics in the area, and when a couple of them stopped by her room on the last day of her life to ask how she was doing, she responded with typical wry humour. "Well, boys, I don't think I'll be going to the dance in Judique tonight," she quipped. (Judique is a small village on the island, still known today for its link to traditional Celtic music.)

I was seventy-one years old when my mother died. My dad had died while I was caught up the blur of my first year in elected office, and I hadn't paused long to mark his death. I was there at her side when my mom died, and that felt right. Twenty-two years elapsed between my parents' deaths, and I hope I grew a little more thoughtful and a little more patient in the intervening years. From my perspective, those two-plus decades as an educator, a choir conductor with a purpose, and an international public health advocate were the pinnacles of my career. I wasn't rescuing patients from fire ladders anymore or hanging out with TV stars, but I was part of the effort to "make the world a better place." I blush to use the phrase, but it's still the right one. And if my whole life traced a great circle route that was destined to take me back to my beloved Cape Breton Island, by 2017 or so I was getting ready to take the last step of that journey.

CHAPTER 11

A PRODIGAL SON FINDS A HOME, 2017-2023

THIS WAS THE PLACE WHERE I WANTED TO SETTLE. IT WAS JUST PAST THE SEAL ISLAND Bridge, which crosses the gut of the inland sea known as the Bras d'Or Lake. My home was located on family land on Boularderie Island, beyond—barely—the slope-shouldered mountains of the Cape Breton Highlands. Our tract of densely forested land and its four houses were located just off Highway 5, the "old road" in local parlance, not a ten-minute drive from the bridge. I built my new home at the exact place where a steep hill was about to become a vertical cliff. The home was modest but modern, surrounded by trees and resting on rock with views of the Great Bras d'Or Channel, and beyond the channel, the great Atlantic and infinity. In my mind, this was the "fixed address" I had been yearning to claim since I'd left home for university in 1960.

Cape Breton Island is a traditional place; the community values I absorbed as a boy have endured. The barter economy still thrives—"I'll put a new roof on your house. You put a rebuilt engine in my truck." People look after themselves, and their own, and their neighbours. My younger neighbours, some of whom I knew as kids, offered to help if I should need it, provided it when I did, and wouldn't take a penny for their troubles. Some of them hauled my new fridge into my new home and set it up for me.

Some people in my generation still speak the Gaelic language; some of their grandchildren are learning it. In many ways, the area feels more Scottish than Scotland. I am in some ways a Celtic romantic, a man who owns a kilt and a sporran and all the rest of it, and this place, for me, feels almost like home.

This land also holds memories. My parents lived here in a home I had built for them and with them in 1972. My father, the man I followed to carpentry jobs as a boy with my own miniature tool kit in hand, finished the interior of the house himself once the contractor had framed it in and left it watertight. In 1991, I built myself a suite on the third floor after deciding to run for political office. When I first moved back to Cape Breton in 2020, I was enthralled by the place. If I was visited by memories of my parents, they were the kindest ghosts imaginable.

I oversaw construction of my new home, designing the working guts—the plumbing, heating, ventilation system, and wiring—myself. I consulted an architect to ensure the place had a sense of balance and proportion. I enjoyed a daily exercise regime: a gentle two-mile jog—a fake jog, really—around nearby Dalem Lake. If the jog sometimes became a hike, or the hike felt more like a trudge, I completed two or three loops of the lake instead of one. In colder months, I traced the circular route on snowshoes, stopping along the way to wonder at the deep red of winter sunsets. In whatever season, at whatever pace, I enjoyed my treks around the lake in the pristine country air.

It still got lonely in the woods. When I tired of talking to squirrels, I jumped into the car to visit friends in the area or to take a longer drive to Halifax. The city was a five-hour trip on a good day, a journey that traces a switchback trek over Kellys Mountain, one of the highest in Nova Scotia. Halifax was my magnetic south pole, Cape Breton my northern one. The city was home to Dalhousie University and its medical school, and to the emergency department that Bob Scharf had virtually created from whole cloth in the 1960s and '70s.

Orlando Hung, my very good friend. thought I should move to the city and immerse myself in emergency medicine as a sort of éminence grise, and he wasn't shy about saying so. He and many other colleagues from the world of medicine were eager to welcome me back to a place where the nearest restaurant was across the street and the hospitals were within walking distance if you lived on the peninsula, the oldest part of town. Orlando clearly thought my decision to live on Cape Breton Island, on an isolated piece of property, was romantic at best—and foolhardy regardless.

There was something to his view. In the winter, the perils of the drive over Kellys Mountain included black ice and whiteouts. In summer, you kept an eye out for tourists driving too fast in vehicles too big to negotiate the tight turns just above the Seal Island Bridge. Still, I loved the drive between city and country, and the destination at each end. A global traveller all my adult life, I enjoyed the solitude of solo driving in North America. As a boy of fourteen, an unlicensed delinquent, I had driven around Sydney Harbour to the great steel city itself (the Sydney steel mill has since closed). During my medical school years, I got my first car—one in a long series of used jalopies—and raced home from Halifax whenever time permitted. In Neils Harbour, where I first practised medicine, I spent a lot of time on the highway as I answered house calls in the Highlands. I even stayed behind the wheel after driving off the road and suffering a serious brain injury from which I was fortunate to recover. When I travelled coast-to-coast to LA in 1972, it was in an old Volvo, not a new narrow-body Boeing 727. I also chose to drive from Toronto to Nova Scotia, several times, when I lived briefly in Canada's biggest city in the late 1980s. (Yes, I could have flown.)

At age eighty, the drive to the city began to seem longer, and the trip over Kellys Mountain felt more perilous. Plus, stuff was happening to me—what doctors would call warning signs. The dirt lane down to the home was steep enough that I bought a snow machine (an all-terrain vehicle with bulldozer-style metal tracks) to get up to the highway in winter. I felt it was okay to drive my car down to the house in other seasons. During the autumn of 2022, when I turned eighty, my car slid off the mucky lane in heavy rains. That same autumn, I took a tumble while chasing visiting toddlers around my house, opening a wound on the top of my head. It revealed a growth that might be malignant. (It wasn't.) I was still handy in a way, competent with a saw or a hammer or a plumb line, and I could still fix things around the house—as my father had done so many years ago. But whether I should have been imitating Bob the Builder at eighty is another question. In the 2021–2022 winter, I banged my head up pretty good trying to do some plumbing outdoors in sub-zero weather. In Halifax that same winter, I hit my head when I slipped on an icy sidewalk after having breakfast with my old friend Orlando at the downtown pancake restaurant where I used to hold court when I was minister of health.

I also had some health problems. Let's face it: they are constant companions as we travel down that one-way street called old age. I was diagnosed in the fall of 2021 with a form of leukemia that would have killed me in short order twenty years earlier. Happily, treatments had advanced. My hematologist in Sydney prescribed a new oral chemo medication that she said should arrest the "progress of the disease"—a medical oxymoron if ever there was one—and keep me alive to a normal old age. (Truth is, I was already approaching the average age of death among Canadian males.)

Over the Christmas season in 2022, it all took a turn for the worse. I found myself stranded at home—down the hill, atop the cliff—with debilitating fatigue. It eased after a few days, but not before Orlando had persuaded me to get into my car and drive to Halifax. By the time I arrived, he'd found a place for me to live—the empty penthouse condo belonging to Mike Murphy, the friend and colleague I had dragooned into leading EHS reform in the 1990s, who was away for the winter in some sunny place. I arrived in Halifax with nothing but the clothes on my back, some spare underwear, medications, a toothbrush, and a bar of soap. I've never been much of a clothes horse and have always been frugal to a fault, so off I went to my favourite haberdasher—Walmart—to buy a pair of pants.

I worked with a lawyer and a financial advisor to figure out my estate. I had once planned to leave the Cape Breton land and houses in a trust fund that would operate the property as a rural retreat for paramedics and other medical professionals after I was among the dearly departed. Now I had to sell the property to afford life in the city. Why would a single doctor need money after decades of practice? Well, I'd given most of it away to the Dalhousie Medical Research Foundation in 2017.[122] At that time I was conscious of the legacy I would leave behind, and my contribution to Dalhousie felt like part of a rounding out of my life. I was in good health but conscious that my time was limited, if not short. In addition, I seemed to be congenitally incapable of accumulating wealth. Mike Murphy once explained this character trait by telling a mutual friend, "Ron is allergic to money."

This all went back to my parents' example and Calvinist instructions. For them, as for me, there was something unseemly about either getting rich or drawing attention to yourself. If you're asking yourself why a man with those values would write a memoir, I'd say that's a good question. Here's the answer. Through the practice of emergency, trauma, and pre-hospital medicine, we can save, enrich, and occasionally prolong lives. I wanted to and still want to tell the world that you can build a great career—and better still, you can lead a useful life—by delivering emergency care in the street, or working beside a hospital stretcher, or exploring in a research lab, or speaking at a United Nations conference. This is the work that absorbed me and absorbs me still.

I was even caught up in the allure of emergency medicine—its magic—as a boy in the 1950s when I used to carry my dad's first aid kit to baseball games in Sydney Mines. Like many older people looking back on their childhoods, I remember mine as special. For a few summers, I was left for a few weeks in the care of my Uncle Tom MacLellan (my mom's brother) and his wife, Joy (née Publicover), who lived in Halifax's historic Hydrostone area—only a few blocks from Mike Murphy's condo, where I stayed in early 2023. Back in the early 1950s, Halifax seemed like the shining city on the hill—modern, sophisticated, and cultured. Aunt Joy, who was eccentric and not inclined to care for me to my mother's standards of oversight and support, often packed me into the car to go on shopping expeditions. I was awestruck by the new Simpsons department store building on Mumford Road, which had opened in 1952. It featured "moving staircases"—to me, a marvel. I spent most of my time on those shopping excursions riding up and down on the escalators while Joy looked for bargains. (I had more fun, and it didn't cost anything.)

I mention my aunt and uncle because returning to Halifax (for the second-last time) in February of 2023 felt like another step in what theologians sometimes call "the great circle of life." (I was in no hurry for it to close completely.) While writing this book, I reconnected with many friends—some in person, many in my memory, more by email and video link. I'll call them "loved ones" just this once, in violation of the Calvinist code in which I was weaned. I met several times with my old college chum Walter Borden—a small, wiry man with a stage voice strong enough to reach the heavens, and with principles held bravely enough to transform him into a lifelong advocate of human rights. I connected with my Acadia University friends Karen MacDonald and Brita Stolz, as brilliant and beautiful now as they were then. I recalled the rapscallion company of Michael Moles and Peter Baskett, smoking and drinking into early evenings and long nights in Hong Kong and

Brighton. I sensed the posthumous scrutiny of the dour John Savage, a man both stern and kind—at least with me. I spoke regularly by phone with my oldest and closest friend—my sister, Donalda. This list could go on and on, but I'm not the sort of man to get weepy in public—or in private.

Truth is, I don't feel weepy despite it all, including the fact that my leukemia took a turn for the worse by the spring of 2023, morphing into a more complex disease requiring aggressive and punishing chemo. I had decided by then to return to Halifax for good but returned to Cape Breton that summer to sell my property and undergo the first stages of my chemo treatments. It felt good to be an Island resident again, if only for a short time. At the cancer clinic in Sydney, I was poked and prodded in a good way (that is, administered chemo) in a comfy reclining chair in a big room full of cancer patients who had the option of closing the curtains around their misery. None ever did, and neither did I. It's considered uppity in the extreme to cut yourself off from your fellow human beings on the Island, even in the cancer clinic. Cape Breton's a great place for company, and you might as well bask in the circle of social warmth (and scrutiny).

By the end of the summer of 2023, I was ready to return to the city for good. In the end, the realist in me got the better of the stubborn and sentimental Celt—who, to be honest, was starting to feel a little tiresome to me. Three blows to the head and a cancer diagnosis should be enough to get any man with means to shift from a splendid rural retreat to an urban apartment. In early September, my Cape Breton neighbour Donnie Patterson, from whose family I had purchased our family land on Boularderie Island half a century earlier, parked a trailer outside my home. He hadn't spoken to me about his purpose, but I understood the Island code—he was helping me move to Halifax. On September 10, he hitched the trailer to his truck and delivered it all to the city, where Orlando had organized a multinational and multilingual crew of box-bearers to take my worldly possessions to my new apartment. On September 11, I drove my 2022 Hyundai Venue—packed to the roof—to Halifax. Within a few weeks, my real estate agent called to say the Cape Breton properties were all sold—which was quite a relief.

I set up digs in a small apartment—inside the Northwood complex that meets my immediate needs and offers "graduated care" if I need it. (Like most people, I hope I won't.) A simple apartment suits me fine. I've been slowly going through the box of mystery files that has trailed me, unopened, from LA to Pittsburgh to Toronto to Nova Scotia. I make snacks in my apartment and am fed three meals a day—though I wouldn't call them square meals. (A group of friends and colleagues deliver real food to my door, and I am grateful for both the calories and the company.) The institutional meals are bland, but I've been living well enough on hospital cafeteria grub for six decades, and my own cooking is so boring that no one could meet the low standards I've set for myself. (My cooking career began and ended in the 1960s when I lit a gas stove too late, blew myself out the door of a trailer in the woods of New Brunswick, and landed on the tent of a honeymooning couple. Things went downhill from there. It's a long story; I'll spare you the details.)

After LA, Pittsburgh, and Toronto, Halifax feels walkable and friendly. From my apartment, I can stroll to Uncle Tom and Aunt Joy's former home in the Hydrostone, where I spent so many summer weeks as a boy. The area, blue-collar to its core when I was kid, now features trendy restaurants, boutiques, galleries, and coffee shops frequented by boomers, hipsters, and young families. When I am up to it, I can walk to the hospital and university district, or downtown to the harbour-front boardwalk, in forty-five minutes. I like the city and relish every moment there, all the more because I know my leukemia is a terminal illness and time is short. With any luck, I'll get a few hundred more days but not much longer. I am okay with that; I've lived long enough.

Back at Dalhousie I enjoy the company and support of a small army of friends, colleagues, and former students. And—major confession here, accompanied by drumroll—I need help from my urban network of friends. As emeritus professor at the medical school, I still present at Grand Rounds from time to time and am asked to deliver lectures via Zoom to med students abroad. I usually talk about the history of modern emergency medicine (after all, I've lived through most of it), and students usually listen. My primary goal, though, is convincing students that medicine is part art, part science. If you cannot connect with people on a human level, if you cannot show that you care, if you cannot earn trust, your patients will suffer. This is particularly true in emergency medicine, a field in which physicians see so many patients for so short a period of time. The relationship has to be built quickly.

I enjoy visiting the emergency ward at the Halifax Infirmary, where I try not to make a nuisance of myself, and I often hang out at the small office Kirk Magee, chair of the department and a good friend, provides for me. I still like being in the world and in the mix.

In short, within weeks of arriving in Nova Scotia's capital city, it was starting to feel like the place where I belonged. And if I really was a prodigal son, Halifax was the home to which I had returned.

ACKNOWLEDGEMENTS

FIRST, WE WOULD LIKE TO THANK THE DOZENS OF LIFELONG FRIENDS AND COLLEAGUES with whom we collaborated in completing this project. Reliving a life, in a series of conversations, was a delight—and a necessary one in our effort to tell the truth.

We are particularly grateful to those people—Sue Newhook, Vonda Hayes, Dan Reid, David Dingwall, Rob Rose, Theresa MacNeil, Jim Bickerton, Maureen Meek—who took the time to review this memoir or parts of it. Their feedback was invaluable.

Without the help of staff at the Halifax Public Library, the Cape Breton University Library, and the Nova Scotia Archives, we would never have managed to read those old newspapers on Microfilm rolls, let alone glean information from them.

Angela Mombourquette at Nimbus Publishing asked all the right probing questions in her review of the text and moved mountains to get this memoir into print. We certainly needed Angela's guidance to complete this memoir—this account of a life remembered.

ENDNOTES

1   Brian J. Zink, *Anyone, Anything, Anytime: A History of Emergency Medicine* (Philadelphia: Mosby Elsevier, 2006).

2   Kevin Goodman, "Imagining Doctors: Medical Students and the TV Medical Drama," *AMA Journal of Ethics* (March 2007), journalofethics.ama-assn.org/article/imagining-doctors-medical-students-and-tv-medical-drama/2007-03.

3   Zink, *Anyone, Anything, Anytime*, 146.

4   Robert McIntosh, "The Boys in the Nova Scotian Coal Mines: 1873 to 1923," *Acadiensis* 16, no. 2 (Spring 1987).

5   Christina M. Lamey, "Davis Day Through the Years: A Cape Breton Coalmining Tradition," *Nova Scotia Historical Review*, 16 no. 2 (1996): 23–33.

6   "Princess Pit, Runaway Rake, Sydney Mines, 1938," Nova Scotia Museum of History (website), museumofindustry.novascotia.ca/nova-scotia-industry/nova-scotia-coal-mining-tragedies/cape-breton-county-coalfield/princess-pit.

7   Pat Devenish, "When War Came to Newfoundland: The Sinking of SS *Caribou*," *Halifax Trident*, November 2, 2020, tridentnewspaper.com/sinking-ss-caribou.

8   Chryssa McAlister and Peter Twohig, "The Check-Off: A Precursor of Medicare in Canada?," *Canadian Medical Association Journal*, cmaj.ca/content/173/12/1504.full.

9   Christopher Moore, "Louisbourg," *The Canadian Encyclopedia* (website), Updated March 2, 2017, thecanadianencyclopedia.ca/en/article/louisbourg.

10   William Davey and Richard MacKinnon, "Nicknaming Patterns and Traditions among Cape Breton Coal Miners," *Acadiensis* 30, no. 2 (Spring 2001).

11   Ronald Stewart, "Referendum Call and Explanation," *Athenaeum* (Acadia University), February 7, 1964.

12   "Algeria Blast Toll Exceeds 100; Port Damage Near $40 Million," *New York Times*, July 26, 1964.

13   Jean-Francois Kahn, "The Bône Explosion Would Have Caused the Death of More than 200 People," *Le Monde*, July 27, 1964. lemonde.fr/archives/article/1964/07/27/l-explosion-de-bone-au-rait-cause-la-mort-de-plus-de-deux-cents-personnes-la-presse-lo-cale-emet-l-hypothese-d-un-sabotage_3051535_1819218.html.

14   "Building Our Department," Department of Medical Neuro-science, Dalhousie University (website), 2023, medicine.dal.ca/departments/department-sites/medical-neuroscience/about/his-tory-of-the-department/mid-20th-century.html.

15   "Interview: Dr. Ron Stewart," *Canadian Parliamentary Review* 17, no. 1 (Spring 1994), revparl.ca/english/issue.asp?art=993&param=148.

16   "Fifty Years of *Emergency!* on Television," Los Angeles County Fire Museum (website), lacountyfiremuseum.com/aug-emergencys-50th.

17   *Code Black—A Look into America's Busiest ER*, directed by Ryan McGarry (CA: Long Shot Factory, 2013).

18 David Ferrell, "Beneath the Hospital, a Bewildering Labyrinth," *Los Angeles Times*, June 28, 2021, latimes.com/archives/la-xpm-2001-jun-28-me-16012-story.html.

19 Zink, *Anyone, Anything, Anytime*, 119.

20 Zink, *Anyone, Anything, Anytime*, 124.

21 "Board of Supervisors," County of Los Angeles, lacounty.gov.

22 National Academy of Sciences and National Research Council, *Accidental Death and Disability: The Neglected Disease of Modern Society* (Washington: National Academies Press, 1966), doi. org/10.17226/9978.

23 Zink, *Anyone, Anything, Anytime*, 152.

24 Ronald D. Stewart, "Dr. Frank Pantridge—Father of Modern EMS?" *Canadian Paramedicine* (March 2017).

25 Stewart, "Dr. Frank Pantridge."

26 J. F. Pantridge and J. S. Geddes, "A Mobile Intensive-Care Unit in the Management of Myocardial Infarction, *Lancet* 290, no. 7510 (Aug. 5, 1967): 271.

27 G. F. Gearty, N. Hickey, G. J. Bourke, and R. Mulcahy, "Pre-hospital Coronary Care Service," *British Medical Journal* 3, no. 5765 (July 3, 1971).

28 Rob Lawrence, "The History of Our History: 50 Years of Prehospital Medicine," EMS1 (podcast), July 14, 2014, ems1. com/historical/articles/the-history-of-our-history-50-years-of-pre-hospital-medicine-PtpkVT0EtxOCKoJv/.

29 Connie Holland, "Reality Plus Drama Equals *Emergency!*," National Museum of American History (website), Sept. 8, 2015, americanhistory.si.edu/blog/reality-plus-drama-equals-emergency.

30 "The Club of Mainz (1983)," *Prehospital and Disaster Medicine* (Cambridge University Press, 2012).

31 "PSA Flight 182," This Day in Aviation: Important Dates in Aviation History (website), thisdayinaviation.com/tag/psa-flight-182.

32 Mark Pinsky, "Doctor Guilty in the 1970 Murder of Wife and Children," *New York Times*, August 30, 1979.

33 Jeanne Lenzer, "Peter Josef Safar: The Father of Cardiopulmonary Resuscitation," *British Medical Journal* 327, no. 7415 (September 2003): 624, ncbi.nlm.nih.gov/pmc/articles/PMC194106.

34 Elaine Schmidt, "In Memoriam: Dr. Gerald S. Levey, 84, Oversaw Building of Ronald Reagan UCLA Medical Center," UCLA Newsroom (website), June 29, 2021, newsroom.ucla.edu/stories/in-memoriam-gerald-levey-ronald-reagan-ucla-medical-center.

35 Bob Retchko, "Suddenly, Bridge Shifts and Nightmare Begins," *Pittsburgh Press*, May 24, 1978, A2.

36 Dolores Frederick, "Pain, Danger on the Bridge Recalled," *Pittsburgh Press*, May 24, 1978, A1.

37 Center for Emergency Medicine of Western Pennsylvania (website), centerem.org.

38 Freedom House of Pittsburgh (website), freedomhousedoc.com.

39 EMS1 and NEMSMA, "How Pittsburgh's 'Freedom House' Shaped Modern EMS Systems," EMS1 (website), January 29, 2019, ems1.com/ems-education/articles/how-pittsburghs-freedom-house-shaped-modern-ems-systems-luEDCMzLZL8XfbzU.

40 Tom Long, "Nancy Caroline, Paramedic Textbook Pioneer Dies at 58," *Boston Globe*, December 13, 2002.

41 "Peter Safar," Lemelson-MIT (website), lemelson.mit.edu/resources/peter-safar.

42   Matthew L. Edwards, "Pittsburgh's Freedom House Ambulance Service: The Origins of Emergency Medical Services and the Politics of Race," *Journal of the History of Medicine and Allied Sciences* 74, no. 4 (October 2019): 455.

43   Peter Hart, "Obituary, Thomas P. Detre," *University Times* (University of Pittsburgh), October 14, 2010, utimes.pitt.edu/archives/?p=13669.

44   "Freedom House: Documentary Tells the Story of the Nation's First Paramedics—Trained by Pitt Physicians," *Pitt Chronicle* (University of Pittsburgh), January 29, 2007, chronicle.pitt.edu/story/freedom-house-documentary-tells-story-nation%E2%80%99s-first-parameics%E2%80%94trained-pitt-physicians.

45   "Henry T. Bahnson, MD, 1920–2003," *Annals of Surgery* 237, no. 4 (2003).

46   "Thomas E. Starzl, MD, PhD, 'Father of Transplantation,' Dies at 90," University of Pittsburgh Medical Center (website), March 5, 2017, upmc.com/media/news/starzl-obit.

47   David McCumber, "Pulitzer Prize Winner, former P-I Reporter Andrew Schneider Dies at 74," *Seattle Times*, February 18, 2017, seattletimes.com/seattle-news/obituaries/pulitzer-prize-winner-andrew-schneider-dies-at-74.

48   McCumber, "Pulitzer Prize Winner."

49   Andrew Schneider, "Medics Bury Fallen Friend," *Pittsburgh Press*, August 27, 1986.

50   "English Football Clubs Banned from Europe," History (website), June 2, 1985, history.com/this-day-in-history/english-football-clubs-banned-from-europe.

51 Dominic Harris, "Margaret Thatcher's Government Thought Football Fans so Violent She Set Up a 'War Cabinet,'" *Independent,* February 19, 2016, independent.co.uk/news/uk/politics/margaret-thatcher-s-government-thought-football-fans-so-violent-she-set-up-a-war-cabinet-a6883226.html.

52 Amy Tikkanen, "Hillsborough Disaster." *Encyclopedia Britannica* (website), June 4, 2023, britannica.com/event/Hillsborough-disaster.

53 "Hillsborough: The Report of the Hillsborough Independent Panel," *The Stationery Office,* September 12, 2012, assets.publishing.service.gov.uk/government/uploads/system/uploads/attachment_data/file/229038/0581.pdf.

54 Jacqueline Gilhooley, "Hillsborough Stories: John-Paul Gilhooley," BBC News (website), April 24, 2014, bbc.com/news/uk-england-27150365.

55 Katy Wheeler, "Touching Tributes to 183 Children Killed in Victoria Hall Disaster as Crisis Fails to Stop Sunderland Remembering," *Sunderland Echo,* June 17, 2020, sunderlandecho.com/news/people/touching-tributes-to-183-children-killed-in-victoria-hall-disaster-as-crisis-fails-to-stop-sunderland-remembering-2886887.

56 Edward Butts, "Dave Williams," *The Canadian Encyclopedia* (website), June 13, 2023, thecanadianencyclopedia.ca/en/article/dave-williams.

57 Ronald D. Stewart and R. Tudor Williams, "Transillumination of the Trachea with a Lighted Stylet," *Anesthesia & Analgesia,* 1986.

58 Ronald D. Stewart, "Tactile Orotracheal Intubation," *Annals of Emergency Medicine* 13, no. 3 (March 1984).

59 Julie Zaztman, "Doctor Helps Avert Disaster," *Halifax Chronicle Herald,* June 1, 1989, 1.

60   Jim Meek, "Savage Takes the Huskilson Test, and Flunks," *Halifax Chronicle Herald*, 1993.

61   Bart Armstrong, "Interview: Dr. Ron Stewart, MLA," *Canadian Parliamentary Review*, January 1994. revparl.ca/english/issue. asp?art=993&param=148.

62   Peter Clancy, James Bickerton, Rodney Haddow, and Ian Stewart, *The Savage Years: The Perils of Reinventing Government in Nova Scotia* (Halifax: Formac, 2000), 32.

63   Parker Donham, "Barrow, MacFadden and 'Suitcase' Simpson: The Final Chapter," *Contrarian* (blog), October 20, 2009, contrarian.ca/2009/10/20/toll-gating/.

64   Leonard Preyra, "Tele-Conventions and Party Democracy: The 1992 Nova Scotia Liberal Leadership Convention," *Canadian Parliamentary Review*, September 14, 2020, revparl.ca/english/ issue.asp?param=147&art=977.

65   "John Savage," *London Telegraph*, May 23, 2003, telegraph.co.uk/ news/obituaries/1430857/John-Savage.html.

66   Julie Collins, "Northside Doctor to Head US Healthcare Task Force," *Cape Breton Post,* February 27, 1993, 1.

67   Lieutenant-Governor Lloyd Crouse, Nova Scotia, Legislature Debates (Hansard), September 13, 1993, 0-nsleg--edeposit-gov-ns-ca.legcat.gov.ns.ca/deposit/HansardDeposit/56-01/19930913. pdf.

68   Governor General of Canada, "Dr. Ronald Daniel Stewart," accessed August 25, 2023, gg.ca/en/honours/recipients/146-4826.

69   Cathy Nicoll, "NDP Demands Stewart's Resignation," *Cape Breton Post,* October 8, 1993, 4.

70   Sharon Montgomery, "Restless Grits Questioning Stewart's Absenteeism," *Cape Breton Post*, December 1, 1993, 6.

71   Sharon Montgomery, "Health Minister Jeered," *Cape Breton Post*, May 16, 1994, 1.

72   Betsy Chambers, "Stewart's Residence Ransacked," Thomson News Service, May 16, 1994.

73   Clancy et al., *The Savage Years*, 80.

74   Editorial, "Human Touch Ends a Protest," *Cape Breton Post*, September 22, 1993, 4.

75   Graeme Hamilton, "Sydney's Tar Ponds: A Deadly Legacy," *Southam News*, February 17, 1997.

76   John Holm, Nova Scotia Legislature Debates, September 23, 1993, 0-nsleg--edeposit-gov-ns-ca.legcat.gov.ns.ca/deposit/Hansard Deposit/56-01/19930923.pdf.

77   Ronald Stewart, Nova Scotia Legislature Debates, September 23, 1993, 0-nsleg--edeposit-gov-ns-ca.legcat.gov.ns.ca/deposit/ HansardDeposit/56-01/19930923.pdf.

78   Clancy et al., *The Savage Years*, 65.

79   Nicoll, "NDP Demands."

80   Mary Clancy, House of Commons Debates, January 27, 1994, ourcommons.ca/DocumentViewer/en/35-1/house/sitting-9/ hansard.

81   André Picard, "The Krever Inquiry," *The Canadian Encyclopedia* (website), accessed August 25, 2023, thecanadianencyclopedia. ca/en/article/krever-inquiry.

82   Horace Krever, *Commission of Inquiry on the Blood System in Canada, final report*, Government of Canada, 1997, publications. gc.ca/site/eng/9.698032/publication.html.

83   Carolyn Ray, "AIDS Advocate Janet Conners Remembered as a Voice 'Impossible to Ignore,'" CBC News (website), August 23, 2022, cbc.ca/news/canada/nova-scotia/aids-advocate-janet-con-ners-remembered-as-a-voice-impossible-to-ignore-1.6558941.

84 Nicoll, "NDP Demands."

85 Nicoll, "NDP Demands."

86 Montgomery, "Health Minister Jeered."

87 Montgomery, "Health Minister Jeered."

88 Liberal Party of Nova Scotia. "Liberal Health Policy," 1993.

89 Jeffrey J. MacLeod, "Healthcare Reform in Nova Scotia: A Study in Pressure Group Politics, 1993–1996," (MA thesis, University College of Cape Breton, 1997), 59.

90 Jennifer Henderson, "Emergency!," *Dalhousie Alumni Magazine* (Fall 1991).

91 Medical Society of Nova Scotia, "It's 3 A.M....Who's Called In to Perform Emergency Surgery?" *Halifax Mail Star*, November 16, 1994, A7.

92 Henderson, "Emergency!," 15.

93 Mike Murphy and Ann Petley-Jones, *Report: Emergency Medical Services Nova Scotia* (Government of Nova Scotia, April 1994).

94 Murphy and Petley-Jones, *Report*, 19.

95 Murphy and Petley-Jones, *Report*, 19.

96 Mike Murphy, "Interview with Jeffrey J. MacLeod," cited in *Healthcare Reform in Nova Scotia*, 77.

97 Murphy, "Interview with Jeffrey J. MacLeod."

98 MacLeod, "Healthcare Reform in Nova Scotia," 79.

99 MacLeod, "Healthcare Reform in Nova Scotia," 7.

100 Clancy et al., *The Savage Years*, 127.

101 Ronald Stewart, Nova Scotia, Legislature Debates, April 23, 1994, nslegislature.ca/legislative-business/hansard-debates/assembly-56-session-2.

102 Clancy et al., *The Savage Years*, 127.

103 *RJR-MacDonald Inc. v. Canada*, [1995] 3 SCR 199, scc-csc.lexum. com/scc-csc/scc-csc/en/item/1290/index.do.

104 David Dingwall, "The Tobacco Control Act, 1997," The MacEachen Institute for Public Policy, Dalhousie University (website), September 27, 2017, dal.ca/dept/maceachen-institute/ events/policy_matters/tobacco_control_act.html.

105 Dingwall expressed his views on my role in supporting the legislation in conversations with Jim Meek in the summer of 2023.

106 K. S. Kendler, J. Myers, M. I. Damaj, and X. Chen, "Early Smoking Onset and Risk for Subsequent Nicotine Dependence: A Monozygotic Co-Twin Control Study," *American Journal of Psychiatry*, April 2013.

107 Rob Cunningham, *Smoke & Mirrors, The Canadian Tobacco War* (Ottawa: International Research Development Centre, 1996), 141.

108 Cunningham, *Smoke & Mirrors*, 142.

109 Cunningham, *Smoke & Mirrors*, 142.

110 D. R. Austin, M. McBurney, M. Kieran, D. Lindsay, and T. Greenaway, "A New Low in Corporate Thuggery," *Globe and Mail*, May 18, 1994, A21, quoted in Cunningham, *Smoke & Mirrors*.

111 Steven J. Rottman, "The World Association for Emergency and Disaster Medicine: Origins, Present Status, and Future Directions," *Prehospital and Disaster Medicine* 6, no. 2 (April-June 1991).

112 "World Congress Backs Canadian Landmine Initiative," Dalhousie University, Faculty of Medicine (website), October 3, 1997.

113 Peter Baskett and Judith Fisher, "T. Michael Moles: A Life to be Celebrated," *Prehospital and Disaster Medicine* 16, no. 2 (April-June 2001).

114 The opening scene in John le Carré's 1977 novel *The Honourable Schoolboy* is set in the Hong Kong's Foreign Correspondents' Club.

115 "Obituary: Peter Baskett," *Guardian*, June 13, 2008, theguardian.com/society/2008/jun/13/nhs.health1.

116 "World Association Backs Nairobi Declaration on Landmine Ban," World Association for Disaster and Emergency Medicine (website), May 20, 2005.

117 Ronald D. Stewart, "Anti-Personnel Landmines: The Next Bold Step...," *Prehospital and Disaster Medicine* 13, no. 2–4 (April-December 1998).

118 Dean Jobb, "A Man of Bold Vision," *Halifax Chronicle Herald*, May 14, 2003, A8.

119 Mary Jane Hampton, "A Rough Road, but a Worthwhile Journey," *Halifax Daily News*, May 5, 2003, 14.

120 "T. Jock Murray, MD," Canadian Medical Hall of Fame (website), cdnmedhall.ca/laureates/jockmurray.

121 "T. Jock Murray, MD," Canadian Medical Hall of Fame.

122 "Dr. Ronald Stewart Makes $1.3-Million Pledge to Dalhousie Medical Research Foundation," *Dal News*, November 3, 2017, dal.ca/news/2017/11/03/dr--ronald-stewart-makes--1-3-million-pledge-to-dalhousie-medica.html.

BIBLIOGRAPHY

"Algeria Blast Toll Exceeds 100; Port Damage Near $40 Million." *New York Times*, July 26, 1964.

Armstrong, Bart. "Interview: Dr. Ron Stewart, MLA." Canadian Parliamentary Review, January 1994. revparl.ca/english/issue. asp?art=993&param=148.

Baskett, Peter, and Judith Fisher. "T. Michael Moles: A Life to be Celebrated." *Prehospital and Disaster Medicine* 16, no. 2 (April-June 2001): 73–74.

Beck, J. Murray. *Politics of Nova Scotia Volume Two 1896–1988.* Tantallon, NS: Four East Publications, 1988.

"Building Our Department." Department of Medical Neuroscience, Dalhousie University (website), 2023. medicine.dal.ca/departments/ department-sites/medical-neuroscience/about/history-of-the-depart-ment/mid-20th-century.html.

Butts, Edward. "Dave Williams." *The Canadian Encyclopedia* (web-site), June 13, 2023. thecanadianencyclopedia.ca/en/article/ dave-williams.

Chambers, Betsy. "Stewart's Residence Ransacked." *Thomson News Service*, May 16, 1994.

Clancy, Peter, James Bickerton, Rodney Haddow, and Ian Stewart. *The Savage Years: The Perils of Reinventing Government in Nova Scotia.* Halifax: Formac, 2000.

Clarke, Sam. "Deaths from Landmines Are on the Rise—and Clearing Them All Will Take Years." *The Conversation* (website), November 15, 2021. theconversation.com/deaths-from-landmines-are-on-the-rise-and-clearing-them-all-will-take-decades-171848.

"The Club of Mainz (1983)." *Prehospital and Disaster Medicine.* Cambridge University Press, 2012.

Collins, Julie. "Northside Doctor to Head US Healthcare Task Force." *Cape Breton Post,* February 27, 1993.

Crouse, Lloyd (Lieutenant-Governor). Nova Scotia Legislature Debates (Hansard), September 13, 1993. 0-nsleg--edeposit-gov-ns-ca.legcat. gov.ns.ca/deposit/HansardDeposit/56-01/19930913.pdf.

Cunningham, Rob. *Smoke & Mirrors, The Canadian Tobacco War.* Ottawa: International Research Development Centre, 1996.

Davey, William, and Richard MacKinnon. "Nicknaming Patterns and Traditions among Cape Breton Coal Miners." *Acadiensis* 30, no. 2 (Spring 2001): 71–83.

Devenish, Pat. "When War Came to Newfoundland: The Sinking of SS Caribou." *Halifax Trident,* November 2, 2020.

"Diana Championed the Ban on Landmines." *Humanity & Inclusion* (website), August 30, 2022. humanity-inclusion.org.uk/en/news/diana-championed-the-ban-of-landmines-25-years-on-from-her-death-their-use-is-on-the-rise-again.

Dingwall, David. "The Tobacco Control Act, 1997." *MacEachen Institute for Public Policy, Dalhousie University* (website), September 27, 2017. scc-csc.lexum.com/scc-csc/scc-csc/en/item/1290/index.do.

"Doctors Debate Landmines." *The Times of London High Education Supplement*, October 13, 1997. timeshighereducation.com/news/doctors-debate-landmines/104086.article.

Donham, Parker. "Barrow, MacFadden and 'Suitcase' Simpson: The Final Chapter." *Contrarian* (blog), October 20, 2009. contrarian.ca/2009/10/20/toll-gating/.

"Dr. Ronald Stewart Makes $1.3-Million Pledge to Dalhousie Medical Research Foundation." *Dal News*, November 3, 2017. dal.ca/news/2017/11/03/dr--ronald-stewart-makes--1-3-million-pledge-to-dalhousie-medica.html.

Edwards, Matthew L. "Pittsburgh's Freedom House Ambulance Service: The Origins of Emergency Medical Services and the Politics of Race." *Journal of the History of Medicine and Allied Sciences* 74, no. 4 (October 2019): 455.

EMS1 and NEMSMA. "How Pittsburgh's 'Freedom House' Shaped Modern EMS Systems." *EMS1* (website), January 29, 2019. ems1.com/ems-education/articles/how-pittsburghs-freedom-house-shaped-modern-ems-systems-luEDCMzLZL8XfbzU.

"English Football Clubs Banned from Europe." *History* (website), June 2, 1985. history.com/this-day-in-history/english-football-clubs-banned-from-europe.

Ferrell, David. "Beneath the Hospital, a Bewildering Labyrinth." *Los Angeles Times*, June 28, 2021. latimes.com/archives/la-xpm-2001-jun-28-me-16012-story.html.

Frederick, Dolores. "Pain, Danger on the Bridge Recalled." *Pittsburgh Press*, May 24, 1978.

"Freedom House: Documentary Tells the Story of the Nation's First Paramedics—Trained by Pitt Physicians." *Pitt Chronicle* (University of Pittsburgh), January 29, 2007. chronicle.pitt.edu/story/freedom-house-documentary-tells-story-nation%E2%80%99s-first-paramedics%E2%80%94trained-by-pitt-physicians.

Gaudet, Charmaine. "Making a Dream Come True in Niger." *Dalhousie: The Alumni Magazine*, Fall 2004.

Gearty, G. F., N. Hickey, G. J. Bourke, and R. Mulcahy. "Pre-hospital Coronary Care Service." *British Medical Journal* 3, no. 5765 (July 3, 1971): 33–35.

Geddes, John S., Ronald D. Stewart, and Thomas F. Baskett. "Evolution of Pre-Hospital Emergency Care: Belfast and Beyond." *Clinical Press*, 2017.

Gilhooley, Jacqueline. "Hillsborough Stories: John-Paul Gilhooley." *BBC News* (website), April 24, 2014. bbc.com/news/uk-england-27150365.

Goodman, Kevin. "Imagining Doctors: Medical Students and the TV Medical Drama." *AMA Journal of Ethics* 9, no. 3 (March 2007): 182–187.

Goodwin, Doris Kearns. Wait Till Next Year: A Memoir. New York: Simon & Schuster, 1997.

Governor General of Canada. "The Honorable Dr. Ronald Daniel Stewart," accessed August 25, 2023. gg.ca/en/honours/recipients/146-4826.

Hamilton, Graeme. "Sydney's Tar Ponds: A Deadly Legacy." *Southam News*, February 17, 1997.

Hampton, Mary Jane. "A Rough Road, but a Worthwhile Journey." *Halifax Daily News*, May 5, 2003.

Harris, Dominic. "Margaret Thatcher's Government Thought Football Fans So Violent She Set Up a 'War Cabinet.'" *Independent,* February 19, 2016. independent.co.uk/news/uk/politics/margaret-thatcher-s-government-thought-football-fans-so-violent-she-set-up-a-war-cabinet-a6883226.html.

Hart, Peter. "Obituary: Thomas P. Detre." *University Times* (University of Pittsburgh), October 14, 2010. utimes.pitt.edu/archives/?p=13669.

Henderson, Jennifer. "Emergency!" *Dalhousie Magazine* 8, no. 1 (Fall 1991): 15–17.

"Henry T. Bahnson, MD, 1920–2003," *Annals of Surgery* 237, no. 4 (April 2003): 591–592.

"Hillsborough: The Report of the Hillsborough Independent Panel." *The Stationery Office*, September 12, 2012. assets.publishing.service.gov.uk/government/uploads/system/uploads/attachment_data/file/229038/0581.pdf.

Holland, Connie. "Reality Plus Drama Equals *Emergency!*," *National Museum of American History* (website), Sept. 8, 2015. americanhistory.si.edu/blog/reality-plus-drama-equals-emergency.

"Interview: Dr. Ron Stewart." *Canadian Parliamentary Review* 17, no. 1 (Spring 1994). revparl.ca/english/issue.asp?art=993&param=148.

Jobb, Dean. "A Man of Bold Vision." *Halifax Chronicle Herald*, May 14, 2003.

"John Savage." *London Telegraph*, May 23, 2003. telegraph.co.uk/news/obituaries/1430857/John-Savage.html.

Kahn, Jean-Francois. "The Bône Explosion Would Have Caused the Death of More than 200 People." *Le Monde*, July 27, 1964. lemonde.fr/archives/article/1964/07/27/l-explosion-de-bone-aurait-cause-la-mort-de-plus-de-deux-cents-personnes-la-presse-locale-emet-l-hypothese-d-un-sabotage_3051535_1819218.html.

Kendler, K. S., J. Myers, M. I. Damaj, and X. Chen. "Early Smoking Onset and Risk for Subsequent Nicotine Dependence: A Monozygotic Co-Twin Control Study." *American Journal of Psychiatry*, April 2013.

Krever, Horace. *Commission of Inquiry on the Blood System in Canada, final report.* Government of Canada, 1997. publications.gc.ca/site/eng/9.698032/publication.html.

Lamey, Christina M. "Davis Day Through the Years: A Cape Breton Coalmining Tradition." *Nova Scotia Historical Review* 16, no.2 (1996): 23–33.

Lawrence, Rob. "The History of Our History: 50 Years of Prehospital Medicine." *EMS1* (podcast), July 14, 2014. ems1.com/historical/articles/the-history-of-our-history-50-years-of-prehospital-medicine-PtpkVT0EtxOCKoJv/.

Le Carré, John. *The Honourable Schoolboy*. New York: Pocket Books, 1977.

Lemelson-MIT (website). "Peter Safar." lemelson.mit.edu/resources/peter-safar.

Lenzer, Jeanne. "Peter Josef Safar: The Father of Cardiopulmonary Resuscitation." *British Medical Journal* 327, no. 7415 (September 2003): 624. ncbi.nlm.nih.gov/pmc/articles/PMC194106/.

Liberal Party of Nova Scotia. "Liberal Health Policy." 1993.

Long, Tom. "Nancy Caroline, Paramedic Textbook Pioneer Dies at 58." *Boston Globe*, December 13, 2002.

Los Angeles County Fire Museum (website). "Fifty Years of *Emergency!* on Television," August 2022. lacountyfiremuseum.com/aug-emergencys-50th.

McAlister, Chryssa. *The Check-Off: The First Mandatory Healthcare Insurance System in Canada*, 2003. Radio documentary. dalspace. library.dal.ca/handle/10222/37725.

McCumber, David. "Pulitzer Prize Winner, former P-I Reporter Andrew Schneider Dies at 74." *Seattle Times*, February 18, 2017. seattletimes.com/seattle-news/obituaries/pulitzer-prize-winner-andrew-schneider-dies-at-74.

McGarry, Ryan, dir. *Code Black—A Look into America's Busiest ER*. CA: Long Shot Factory, 2013.

McIntosh, Robert. "The Boys in the Nova Scotian Coal Mines: 1873 to 1923." *Acadiensis* 16, no. 2 (Spring 1987): 35–50.

———. "Canada's Boy Miners." *The Beaver* 67, no. 6 (December 1987–January 1988): 34–38. canadashistoryarchive.ca/canadas-history/the-beaver-dec-1987-jan-1988/flipbook/2/.

MacLeod, Jeffrey J. "Health Care Reform in Nova Scotia: A Study in Pressure Group Politics, 1993–1996." MA thesis, University College of Cape Breton, 1997.

Medical Society of Nova Scotia. "It's 3 A.M....Who's Called In to Perform Emergency Surgery?" *Halifax Mail Star.*

Meek, Jim. "Savage Takes the Huskilson Test, and Flunks." *Halifax Chronicle Herald,* 1993.

Montgomery, Sharon. "Restless Grits Questioning Stewart's Absenteeism." *Cape Breton Post,* December 1, 1993.

———. "Health Minister Jeered." *Cape Breton Post,* May 16, 1994.

Moore, Christoper. "Louisbourg." *The Canadian Encyclopedia* (website). Updated March 2, 2017. thecanadianencyclopedia.ca/en/article/louisbourg.

Murphy, Mike. "Interview with Jeffrey J. MacLeod." Cited in *Healthcare Reform in Nova Scotia.*

Murphy, Mike and Ann Petley-Jones. *Report: Emergency Medical Services Nova Scotia.* Government of Nova Scotia, April 1994.

National Academy of Sciences and National Research Council. *Accidental Death and Disability: The Neglected Disease of Modern Society.* Washington: National Academies Press, 1966. doi.org/10.17226/9978.

Nicoll, Cathy. "NDP Demands Stewart's Resignation." *Cape Breton Post,* October 8, 1993.

Nova Scotia Museum of Industry. "Princess Pit, Runaway Rake, Sydney Mines, 1938." museumofindustry.novascotia.ca/nova-scotia-industry/nova-scotia-coal-mining-tragedies/cape-breton-county-coalfield/princess-pit.

"Obituary: James Francis Frank Pantridge." *British Medical Journal* 330, no. 7494 (April 2, 2005): 793.

"Obituary: Peter Baskett." *Guardian,* June 13, 2008. theguardian.com/society/2008/jun/13/nhs.health1.

Pantridge, J. F., and J. S. Geddes. "A Mobile Intensive-Care Unit in the Management of Myocardial Infarction." *Lancet* 290, no. 7510 (Aug. 5, 1967): 271.

Picard, André. "The Krever Inquiry." *The Canadian Encyclopedia* (website), accessed August 25, 2023. thecanadianencyclopedia.ca/en/article/krever-inquiry.

Pinsky, Mark. "Doctor Guilty in the 1970 Murder of Wife and Children." *New York Times,* August 30, 1979.

Plewa, Michael C., MD, Andrew B. Peitzman, MD, and Ronald D. Stewart, MD. "Benign Cervical Prevertebral Soft Tissue Swelling in Traumatic Asphyxia." *Journal of Trauma* 38, no. 6 (June 1995): 937–940.

Preyra, Leonard. "Tele-Conventions and Party Democracy: The 1992 Nova Scotia Liberal Leadership Convention." *Canadian Parliamentary Review,* September 14, 2020. revparl.ca/english/issue.asp?param=147&art=977.

"PSA Flight 182." *This Day in Aviation: Important Dates in Aviation History* (website). thisdayinaviation.com/tag/psa-flight-182.

"PTI History." *Health Services, Los Angeles County* (website). dhs.lacounty.gov/emergency-medical-services-agency/home/paramedic-training-institute/pti-history.

Ray, Carolyn. "AIDS Advocate Janet Conners Remembered as a Voice 'Impossible to Ignore.'" *CBC News* (website), August 23, 2022. cbc. ca/news/canada/nova-scotia/aids-advocate-janet-conners-remembered-as-a-voice-impossible-to-ignore-1.6558941.

Retchko, Bob. "Suddenly, Bridge Shifts and Nightmare Begins." *Pittsburgh Press*, May 24, 1978.

RJR-MacDonald Inc. v. Canada. 3 SCR [1995]. scc-csc.lexum.com/ scc-csc/scc-csc/en/item/1290/index.do.

Rottman, Steven J. "The World Association for Emergency and Disaster Medicine: Origins, Present Status, and Future Directions." *Prehospital and Disaster Medicine* 6, no. 2 (April-June 1991): 171–174.

Schmidt, Elaine. "In Memoriam: Gerald S. Levey, 84, Oversaw Building of Ronald Reagan UCLA Medical Center." *UCLA Newsroom* (website), June 29, 2021. newsroom.ucla.edu/stories/ in-memoriam-gerald-levey-ronald-reagan-ucla-medical-center.

Schneider, Andrew. "Medics Bury Fallen Friend." *Pittsburgh Press*, August 27, 1986.

"Seat belt." Wikimedia Foundation. Last modified date July 18, 2023. en.wikipedia.org/wiki/Seat_belt.

Stewart, Ronald. "Referendum Call and Explanation." *Athenaeum* (Acadia University), February 7, 1964.

Stewart, Ronald D. "Anti-Personnel Landmines: The Next Bold Step." *Prehospital and Disaster Medicine* 13, no. 2–4 (April-December 1998): 12–15.

———. "Dr. Frank Pantridge—Father of Modern EMS?" *Canadian Paramedicine* (March 2017).

———. "Tactile Orotracheal Intubation." *Annals of Emergency Medicine* 13, no. 3 (March 1984): 175–178.

Stewart, Ronald D. and R. Tudor Williams, "Transillumination of the Trachea with a Lighted Stylet," *Anesthesia & Analgesia,* 1986

"T. Jock Murray, MD." *Canadian Medical Hall of Fame* (website). cdn-medhall.ca/laureates/jockmurray.

"Thomas E. Starzl, MD, PhD, 'Father of Transplantation,' Dies at 90." University of Pittsburgh Medical Center (website), March 5, 2017. upmc.com/media/news/starzl-obit.

Tikkanen, Amy. "Hillsborough Disaster." *Encyclopedia Britannica* (website), June 4, 2023. britannica.com/event/Hillsborough-disaster.

Wheeler, Katy. "Touching Tributes to 183 Children Killed in Victoria Hall Disaster as Crisis Fails to Stop Sunderland Remembering." *Sunderland Echo,* June 17, 2020. sunderlandecho.com/news/people/touching-tributes-to-183-children-killed-in-victoria-hall-disaster-as-crisis-fails-to-stop-sunderland-remembering-2886887.

"World Association Backs Nairobi Declaration on Landmine Ban." *World Association for Disaster and Emergency Medicine* (website), May 20, 2005.

"World Congress Backs Canadian Landmine Initiative." *Dalhousie University, Faculty of Medicine* (website), October 3, 1997.

Zaztman, Julie. "Doctor Helps Avert Disaster." *Halifax Chronicle Herald,* June 1, 1989.

Zink, Brian J. *Anyone, Anything, Anytime: A History of Emergency Medicine.* Philadelphia: Mosby Elsevier, 2006.

INDEX